Praise for Meredith

Triathlon for the Every Woman

"A must-read for anyone who feels tired of living a life with not enough time and way too much drama. This book shines a poignant, down-to-earth and humorous light on your journey to change your life."

—EMILY GIFFIN, *New York Times* bestselling author of *Something Borrowed* and *All We Ever Wanted*

"Meredith writes the gospel for how to get out of your own way. This book is a game-changer for anyone who is ready to face her own, personal Truth."

—KYRSTEN SINEMA, United States Senator for Arizona

"Meredith has an amazing ability to deal with the truth, no matter how it hurts. Her matter-of-fact style and candor hits you directly in the gut and will help you open up to yourself. It is the pain and shame she is able to share in *No Nonsense* that will help you heal your life's wounds."

—MIKE REILLY, voice of IRONMAN and author of *Finding My Voice*

"Meredith Atwood is a woman after my own heart. Her new book cuts to the chase and shows us how to cut out the bullshit in life—starting with ourselves."

—LAUREN ZANDER, life coach, cofounder and chairwoman of Handel Group, creator of Inner.U, and author of *Maybe It's You*

"Meredith Atwood does a fantastic job of calling us out by her own example so we can begin to identify the easy steps to get to the root of our own excuses—these excuses that are holding us back from achieving the health and well-being we all deserve."

—DR. WILL COLE, leading functional medicine expert, IFMCP, DC and author of *The Inflammation Spectrum*

"*The Year of No Nonsense* is part tough love, part a swift kick in the ass, and all amazingly useful. Meredith Atwood is the kind person you want as your BFF—snarky, insightful, genuinely kind. With this book, there's little you can't tackle in life."

—DAVID LEITE, author of *Notes On a Banana:*
A Memoir of Food, Love, and Manic Depression

"Tough, frank, courageous, and fun, *The Year of No Nonsense*, will change your life. It's already changed mine."

—BRIDGET QUINN, author of *Broad Strokes:*
15 Women Who Made Art and Made History (In That Order)

"Atwood is both deeply human and utterly inspiring; reading her book is like spending quality time with your fun, supportive best friend who tells it like it is (but doesn't make you feel bad in the process). She blazes her own path and welcomes us all on her exhilarating journey of self-discovery. With tough love, good humor and unvarnished honesty, Atwood will help you finally take control of your life."

—ERIN CARLSON, author of *I'll Have What She's Having* and *Queen Meryl*

"A raw and refreshing straight shot of truth that will guide you to find where you are settling as a passenger and propel you into the pilot seat of your life."

—RANDY SPELLING, author of *Unlimiting You*

"A kick in the butt and a challenge to face the kind of life you really want to live, *The Year of No Nonsense* helped me begin to see the kind of nonsense I give space to in my own life—and helped me devise a map for picking my way out of it, one piece of nonsense at a time."

—KIM DINAN, author of *The Yellow Envelope*

"In *The Year of No Nonsense*, Meredith Atwood gets real, raw, and honest and shares hard-won insights and advice guaranteed to help everyone begin dealing with—and doing away with—the Nonsense in their own lives."

—JOYCE SHULMAN, CEO Macaroni Kid and 99 Walks

"*The Year of No Nonsense* is going to help a lot of people achieve greater success in sports and life by being a little more real with themselves, not only because it's chockfull of good advice but also because Meredith Atwood walks the talk, being ruthlessly, hilariously, and movingly real with herself throughout the book."

—MATT FITZGERALD, author of *Life is a Marathon*

"There are books that crack the frozen ice of our own willful denial. This one utterly shatters it. You cannot read Meredith Atwood's unvarnished account of confronting her 'nonsense' without having to give your own BS a square look in the face. I found relief, humor, insight, and not a little bit of uneasiness in these pages. And for this, I'm am so very grateful and so very changed."

—SASHA HEINZ, PhD, MAPP, Developmental Psychologist, Positive Psychology Maven, Life Coach, Human

"Meredith's frank, no-nonsense, honest style is refreshing. She lays a path that can be applied day-to-day in relationships at work, at home and when facing big goals or projects! It's clear she is living her message and I love that. Meredith, thank you for offering your journey so transparently to help me and others identify our nonsense and makes choices to life more fully!"

—SUSAN CLARKE, author of *The Beauty of Conflict* and *The Beauty of Conflict for Couples*

THE YEAR OF NO NON-SENSE

How to Get Over Yourself and On with Your Life

MEREDITH ATWOOD

LIFE
LONG

Da Capo Lifelong Books
Hachette Book Group
1290 Avenue of the Americas, New York, NY 10104
www.dacapopress.com
@DaCapoPress

Printed in the United States of America
First Edition: December 2019

Published by Da Capo Lifelong Books, an imprint of Perseus Books, LLC, a subsidiary of Hachette Book Group, Inc. The Da Capo Lifelong Books name and logo is a trademark of the Hachette Book Group.

The Hachette Speakers Bureau provides a wide range of authors for speaking events. To find out more, go to www.hachettespeakersbureau.com or call (866) 376-6591.

The publisher is not responsible for websites (or their content) that are not owned by the publisher.

Print book interior design by Linda Mark.
Onion illustration courtesy of James A. Atwood, IV

Library of Congress Cataloging-in-Publication Data has been applied for.

ISBNs: 978-0-7382-8553-5 (trade paperback); 978-0-7382-8552-8 (ebook)

LSC-C

10 9 8 7 6 5 4 3 2 1

"It takes courage to grow up and become who you really are."
—e. e. cummings

To James and Stella.

Remember to Truly Live YOUR Life. You are Loved.

"When you have something to say, silence is a lie
—and tyranny feeds on lies."

Jordan B. Peterson
12 Rules for Life: An Antidote to Chaos

Contents

NONSENSE*

Self-Sabotage SCARCITY blame Lack of Accountability RAGE
UNWORTHINESS Retail Therapy A Spoon and a Jar of Almond Butter
Covert Abuse Excuses for Anything and Everything SELF-DESTRUCTION
Never Saying No NEVER SAYING YES Depression Self-Hate PROCRASTINATION
Comparison Perfectionism GOSSIP Fear of Being Alone Addiction Bullying
"TOO BUSY" Limiting Ourselves NAME CALLING Bad Table Manners
Refusing to Floss Teeth BALANCE Social Media Rage STRESS EATING
stress not-eating Cheating (on Anything) Frenemies
FAILING TO RETURN STUFF BECAUSE TOO LAZY TO MAIL RACISM
HELICOPTER PARENTING Judgments A Spoon and a Half-Gallon of Ice Cream
PARENTING VICARIOUSLY Porn Addiction Being a Nosy Parker HOARDING STUFF
Shame Emotional Outbursts EXCESS Grudges WASTE Fear of Failure
HATE Fear of Success Fear Chronic Looking on the Dark Side
Being Rude to Customer Service Representatives, Servers, or Transportation Workers
FEAR OF RELAPSE FEAR OF CLOWNS SELF-BLAME No Accountability
BIASES MISOGYNY Overeating as a Habit Emotional Abuse
Drunk Mommy/Daddy Routine LIVING IN THE PAST LIVING ONLY IN THE FUTURE
Lying to Yourself compulsive shopping STALKING Never Going to the Dentist
DRAMA BELIEVING THE WORLD REVOLVES AROUND YOU
Compulsive Buying of Books when 154 Books Sit on Nightstand
doing everything for someone else INDECISIVENESS
A SPOON AND A JAR OF PEANUT BUTTER Hoarding Emotions RUDENESS
Being a Stingy Tipper The Endless Bucket of Popcorn at the Movies
THE ENDLESS SOFT DRINK AT THE MOVIES Trying to Make Everyone Happy
Never Washing Your Face Sticking Head in Sand AFFAIRS
Never Asking for Help SKIPPING THE YEARLY PHYSICAL
Wish/Hope Mentality Obsessing Over Someone(s) on Social Media
NAIL-BITING OVERANALYSIS COMPULSIVE BEHAVIORS Toe-Nail Biting
HOMOPHOBIA Asking the Wrong Questions ABUSE
SKIPPING BATHING FOR AN EXTENDED PERIOD OF TIME WITHOUT GOOD REASON
Bad Socks A Bad Bra BAD SHOES Answering the Wrong Questions
STAYING STUCK No Ownership Seeking Attention EMOTIONAL SPIRALS
Keeping Up with the Joneses (or Kardashians) NEGATIVE SELF-TALK
"Righteous" Anger A Spoon and a Jar of Nutella
Control Issues PERHAPS SPOONS BEING STINGY

*List is not exclusive. List is objective and subjective. My Nonsense is not your
Nonsense. Your Nonsense is not her or his Nonsense. More ahead.

Introduction: Your Time to LIVE

I CAME ACROSS SOME PICTURES THE OTHER DAY, TUCKED AWAY IN A drawer. Photos, discolored by time and hidden in an envelope as if to say, "No one should see what's inside. Like, ever."

Photos of me, standing in my underwear.

Photos taken from the front, the back, and the side. I was holding a newspaper. Clearly a timer had been involved because the photos were off-center, the camera clearly on a chair or a dresser. I wasn't smiling.

Classic "before" pictures.

I squinted at the newspaper in the photos. I couldn't see the date. But I remembered the underwear. Victoria's Secret, circa 1999. I also remembered the room—in my first apartment. My first place in the world that was (sort of) my own.

This "before" picture was beautiful.

Age nineteen. Flawless skin. Boobs pointing more or less upward. A body devoid of stretchmarks. A belly, but nothing that cutting back on the beer could not have "fixed" easily, seamlessly, forgivingly.

My size? *Perfectly healthy.*

My sadness? *Insurmountable.*

My fears? *Tangible.*

Self-loathing? *Deep and endless.*

The path to destruction? *Imminent.*

Substantial pain and trauma? *There it is.* Holy . . .

Back then, the focus of my criticism was "fat." But twenty years later, I notice mostly my eyes. The hollow, pained eyes—the eyes that reflected the foreshadowing of nearly two decades of addiction, suppression of unidentified trauma, pain of disappointment, and fear of the future. The camera lens reflected eyes of anger, maybe even rage.

Only I never saw it that way—until now.

I see it all now, not because I am older or wiser but because hindsight is 20/20, and that's one of Life's greatest bonuses—and downers. We have the luxury of seeing things differently as we age and grow, sure. We have the capacity to remember, to relive, and to experience the pain of the past in new ways.

But merely time passing was not all that allowed me to *see.* After all, time can pass and pass, and we can still remain utterly blind.

Somewhere along the recent way, I stuck a stake in the ground, and I said, "No more. No more of this. No more of ALL of THIS."

This? This what? What is *this*?

I bet you know what I mean, though. Because I had a "this," and you have a "this"—and these are the things that plague us. These are the things, habits and behaviors, gut-sickening feelings that are making us freaking nuts.

"This" has a name: Nonsense.

I see "this" now because I have chosen to embark on a Life of less Nonsense. This Life of less Nonsense began with my experiment that I aptly and obviously dubbed The Year of No Nonsense.

The Year of No Nonsense was not about me curing or fixing or surviving mental illness . . . or addictions . . . or relationships . . . or self-sabotage . . . or trauma. Rather, the Year of No Nonsense was (and is) about what can be done about these (very real, very difficult) things standing in the way of us becoming the best versions of ourselves.

The road to healing or changing the big things—like a bad relationship or even a rotten career—starts with making room for change. We make room for change, for recovery, by seeing the Truth. Once we see the Truth, we create a path. And once on the path, we can begin the process of forward motion. One day, one step at a time.

Here is what I found: most of us are living lives full of Nonsense. Small, silly Nonsense that we can laugh about.

Huge, catastrophic Nonsense that knocks the breath out of our lungs and makes the bile rise in our throat when we remember it, experience it, relive it. Nonsense that's totally our faults; some that is tragically and inexplicably put upon us by someone else's disgusting or ridiculous Nonsense.

"Nonsense" is a lighthearted word for some deep, dark bullshit.

We have so much suffering going on inside us that we don't see the Nonsense for what it is. We don't understand our roles in it either—what is 100 percent our faults or what is 100 percent not our faults. We are wandering. We don't see the Other People, we don't see ourselves. We don't want to see ourselves. We don't want to feel either—not our feelings or our bodies; we want out of it all. We don't recognize ourselves to the point that we choose darkness over light, pain over peace, anger over love, loneliness over forgiveness, and sometimes death over Life. (Again, Nonsense: such a light word for dark stuff.)

Of all the lessons I learned in this process, however, one lesson stands out to me the most: THIS is the Year to Live. In this Year of No Nonsense—starting right now—we are here to Live.

No matter where we came from, what we have experienced, who hurt us (intentionally or not), who tried to break us, we are here to Live. We are here to wake ourselves up, to grab Life and Live. We are here to feel—even the hard things. We are here to embody our bodies, to take up space we are worthy of and be. We can and must feel the emotions. Even those destructive urges toward perfectionism, emotions of unworthiness, failure, and disappointment.

Because we are here to live, we must feel, and we must see. Even when we don't want to feel or see.

The Year of No Nonsense teaches us that we can overcome—even the seemingly impossible. We are here to walk (run) through the pain, prosper, and live with the irreparable cracks. We are not here to fix everything—we are here to thrive despite all the fragile, colorful, and wild fissures—because we are not broken. Despite what the world wants us to believe—we are not broken. And we will not be broken. We are alive. We are powerful. We are strong. *We are here to see; we are here to Live.*

Maybe you are mostly happy and don't see what's so hard about Life, and you're wondering what's so glum. That's okay—and that's great actually. But you can be mostly great and still have Nonsense. (There's also the chance of having completely numbed yourself and your feelings into a state of complacency.) *We are here to Live.*

You picked up this book for a reason. And I will assume that the Universe makes no mistakes. So you and I? We're bonded now. In this Nonsense quest. Welcome.

Look, we don't need sophomore year "before" pictures. We don't need age forty or sixty "before" pictures either. We aren't a "before" now, and we weren't a "before" then.

We are a *now*. One day we will look back on this *now*—even if right now is painful—and we will wish we had been grateful for this moment.

We are *here to Live.*

We can make this the Year that changes everything—starting today. Whether it's January or June, today is the day to reclaim the person you are—the person you were born to be.

The person you *have always been* . . . before Nonsense got in the way.

Stay with me. Stay with you.

This is your time to Live.

This is YOUR Year of No Nonsense.

PART I

GET OVER AND THROUGH THE PAST

1

Start Where You *Were*

NEARING THE END OF 2015, I WAS THIS PSEUDO-INSPIRATIONAL, Z-list social media character—with just enough of an audience to be dangerous. I was a former-fat-still-fat-girl who slogged through triathlons, authored a book, lawyered, and helped people live their best lives.

I was inspirational as fuck.

I was also a bit of a fraud.

After changing my Life "big time" through triathlon and acquiring all sorts of coaching certifications, a growing business, and race finishes, I had ended up in a similar place to when I started the whole shebang—isolated, overweight, tired, sad, and angry—only with "triathlete" and "author" to add to my ever-growing résumé of bullshit.

And worse than that, I knew it.

But actually I had come far from where I *started*—a jiggly, can't-run-a-mile-out-of-shape mom to an IRONMAN finisher. I had built a community and shared my story. I had made some changes. Life became better, but it was like a weird airplane upgrade. I had a seat closer to the front and a few cheap perks, but everything else was still middle seat, economy class, with a crying baby kicking my headrest.

I had upgraded, but I was still suffering. Yes, *suffering*.

And I was suffering in the exact same ways that I had always suffered. My suffering at age thirty-five felt the same as my suffering at age five, fifteen, and twenty-five. *Unworthy. Enormous. Disappointment. Failure. Crazy. Hard to Love.*

I made good money. (So why was I broke?) I worked out all the time. (So why was I still "morbidly obese" according to a chart?) I was a triathlete. (So why did I hate my body?) I had a kind, hardworking husband and two healthy, beautiful kids. (So why did I feel unloved? Unsafe? Unhappy?) *Am I crazy?* became the drumbeat in my head.

On the outside, I was (still) the wife and mom who held it all together. Even when I drank a martini and two bottles of wine and ate a large pizza (after a substantial dinner), I appeared okay. I never said I felt wonderful, but I made Life happen even though I felt miserable, struggled with depression, and wore pants that kept getting tighter and tighter. No matter how destructively the night before had ended, however, I would spring out of bed with the sun, throw on my workout clothes, announce that it was time for school, and drag my hungover, swollen arse to the bus stop with the kids and a death grip on my coffee cup.

I would think to myself, *I got this. I can do this. I will not kill anyone today. I can be nice to this annoying woman on Facebook Messenger (Ding! Ding!). I can smile at the bus stop moms. I can smile. I can smile. I got this. You got this, Meredith.*

I was full of crap. *I gots nothing, Meredith* is what churned in my head. Deep down, I knew the bottom was coming. But I was deep in the River Nile as well.

One particular morning, I saw the bottom.

I got smashed the night before and stayed up too late listening to Tori Amos and wondering what had happened to my *Pretty Good*

Year. When the alarm went off—on a school day—I did something unprecedented: I turned it off, rolled over, and went back to sleep. I did not get dressed for the gym. I did not get the kids ready for school. I did not whisper to my husband an excuse like, "I am sick." I did *nothing.*

I did none of my duties.

Hell had clearly frozen over. I always did the required things, no matter what.

Except on this day, I said, "No."

I said no to Life, to my kids. I said no to my job, my workout, my husband, my responsibilities, the teachers at the school, and everyone. Literally, if Oprah had called me, I would have said no to her too. I pulled my puffy middle finger out from under the covers, shot a massive bird into the air, and said, "Not today, Life. Fuck you."

And I meant it.

A few hours later, I woke up in a sweaty ball of covers, crusty-faced and surprised at the mere experience of waking up. *Where am I? Oh yes. Home sweet crap horrible Life home.* I pulled my heavy body out of bed and slogged downstairs. The desire and need for any workout had vanished. The kids were gone, so I assumed they had made it to school (or were missing)—in that moment I shrugged at either outcome.

I saw a note on the counter.

The note was strategically placed next to two (empty) bottles of unoaked chardonnay, a pint of ice cream (also empty), and (one of the many) overdue credit card bills.

The note contained one line. One sentence, in my husband's bitter, scientific-smartypants handwriting:

 You need to get your shit together.

I blinked. I read. I reread.

I pulled my phone from the dirty back pocket of the sweatpants I had been wearing for a few days (weeks). I began texting the tirade of anger that righteously flies from the fingers of a wronged, amazing wife and mother. I wanted to reach deep into my résumé drawer (not that I have one) and pull out my résumé, text it to my husband, and say, "I am *amazing!* Look at all the things I do! And am! And have done. Look at this! Look at this one! And this! What about this one? Oh, and I do all of these things FOR YOU and THOSE KIDS!"

I was mad—an understatement. I lived with this guy. He was witness to all the things on paper that I was. *And this was what I got? This was the thanks? Harumph.*

I finished composing the longest, angriest text with accompanying violent emojis, and I almost pressed send. But something caught the corner of my eye. It wasn't the downed wine bottles or empty ice cream container. It wasn't the blasted sticky note on the sticky counter.

What caught my eye was a wrinkly, kid-stained poster board. A poster with purple and black marker scrawled across it.

My heart lurched into my throat.

There it was: a first-grade science project that I had promised to help complete that morning. A poster that meant something very important to a very small, yet important person in my Life. I had not only failed to help our daughter finish her project, but I hadn't even gotten out of bed to fake a reason why I couldn't help her.

I didn't bother to show up.

Worse than that, I didn't care.

I was angry, yes. At myself. At the world. But I was most angry at the fact that my husband had called me on the giant greasy bucket of Kentucky fried bullshit I had been selling myself and the world. I wasn't holding myself together—my mind, body, and soul were as if Scotch-taped together by a kindergartner. I was disappointing people left and right. Mostly, myself. I was pretending to be all inspirational—when I was a damn liar and a fake who couldn't even get out of bed on a random weekday.

I had created a mess for myself.

It was all there—before me in black and white, with my foul cactus mouth, poster board, wine bottles, empty Ben & Jerry's, and soggy pizza box. My choices had turned my reality into a real-time frat house: a messy, stinky box of bad beer and worse ideas.

My sour stomach turned on me with a vengeance, and the Truth shined in with the power of a search-and-rescue spotlight. I backspaced the text message. I called in sick to work (as if that was even necessary at 9:30 a.m.), and I began to clean the kitchen.

All of the sudden, I was awake.

And deeply, darkly, and dangerously ashamed.

I could not live this way, not a second longer. I couldn't live with the current bad habits, thoughts, anger, and addictions. I couldn't live with the shame and regret of it either. I couldn't live with the same suffering I had been experiencing year after year, decade after decade, for as long as I could remember. I knew something (else) had to change.

Unfortunately, that something was me.

Which meant, I still had a lot of work ahead of me.

YOUR HOUSE, YOUR RULES

Soon (but not that soon) after the famous sticky-note-pocalypse, I quit drinking.

Step one.

And a year after that, I hightailed it out of the legal profession.

Step two.

Two good and big things—yet I did not seem to have the time or peace I thought I would. Each month without a real and regular paycheck was interesting as well. I wasn't sleeping (no news there). I had made strides with nutrition and body image, but I would still find myself on multiple-day food binges. Loads of resulting self-hate. Destructive cycle. Pain. Suffering.

Another shift began to shimmy and shake. I felt like I was living on a fault line, and the earth was going to crack open and swallow my ass whole. Something (bad) was going to happen—and it was going to rock my Universe. I could sense it. I began to live in a low-boil sense of dread.

I failed to start almost every major sporting race I registered for. My grandmother died—a loss of huge proportions. I experienced major betrayals, epic professional explosions and implosions, failures. I took over a struggling business and sank way too many loans into it, attempting to prop it up. Also, turned out that my friend circle was suddenly shaped more like the Ultimate Fighter Octagon.

I wasn't innocent in all of it either. I did my fair share of fighting (wrongly and rightly). I could have handled things differently. But that's part of the narrative now.

I call this particular time The Year That Can Kiss My Ass.

I realized I was at the bottom of my new bottom. My Life, the fraud, was in need of a complete overhaul. I needed to do something, but wasn't sure what.

During this time, I stayed sober—I had to because there was much, much work to be done. Inside I carried the common theme of struggle. I still wasn't getting it—whatever "it" was. I was missing pieces of something.

What was it?

My world felt like it was closing in. And when I feel like my world is closing in, I make lists.

I made two lists:

Things going well in my Life; and

Things that suck ass.

The Going Well List was unremarkable.

This was not a gratitude list, mind you, but a list of objective things that I believed were going well in my Life: relationships, Health, and career sorts of things. Things that "on paper" I could tick the boxes and say, "Going well. Check."

The list was scary short. I stared at it for a minute.

Then I wrote, in messy scrawl, across the page, "Ripe with Potential." Welp, I thought. *That was short and easy. Let's make another list.*

Across the next page, I scribbled at the top "Things That Suck Ass," and I started writing—the TTSA List.

The main issue I gleaned from my TTSA List was how much time and energy I spent doing things like managing drama, pretending to be friends with people who hated me, and texting people I didn't even like. Also on the list was eating food I didn't like, then eating all the food that I loved and subsequently binged on and hated myself for eating. Giving copious amounts of money to those who never even said thank you—and then shockingly would ask for more. Giving folks my focus and attention and then watching them run over me with it. Saying yes to things and people who zapped energy from me. Taking on projects that I should have said no to from the beginning.

As I looked at the TTSA List, I wondered when the job description for my Life became "pushover," "let me give you something else for free," and "punching bag." I certainly had a responsibility to be kind, to take the high road, to be an example or whatnot. Dude, I worked on that—a major challenge at this stage of my Life. But after several outrageous encounters, I struggled.

I had officially become a diplomatic, people-pleasing, high-road-riding punching bag.

A lot of it came with sobriety too.

When I was drinking, I would fire off my mouth or fingers (on social media) and pretend like I didn't care. As a sober person, I had learned the art of keeping my mouth shut. Because I had so many drunken regrets. But as a *lo siento*, I became gullible, timid, ashamed, and somewhat pretendedly indifferent.

After I made the TTSA List, I felt nothing.

Then I felt everything at once. After reading and rereading my list, I panicked. My TTSA List was huge, and my Life was clearly not going as I had meticulously planned. I was "Ripe with Potential," according to the other list, but yet, I was spiraling.

I took the time to stop and breathe for a hot minute. I looked at the things on the TTSA List and saw the whole list blob together like one of those weird "Magic Eye" posters from the 1990s.

I unfocused my eyes, refocused, unfocused—and BAM. I could see it.

Nonsense.

My TTSA List was a list full of Nonsense. So much smelly, rotten Nonsense. My fault, not my fault, but Nonsense. *Why had I not seen this before? How had I lost track of what mattered to me?*

I immediately sensed, "If I can get rid of the Nonsense on this list, or this whole TTSA List altogether, then I will be able to breathe."

Suddenly, I felt like a kid at Christmas—unwrapping present after present of Nonsense. Everything was revealing itself. Is this Nonsense—yes or no? Is this Nonsense—yes or no? Is this Nonsense—yes or no? So much Nonsense! Perhaps you have seen the YouTube video of a kid unwrapping an avocado for a Christmas present. The moral of the video is that he very politely shows extreme gratitude for his "gift" of an avocado.

He says, all gleefully, "It's an avocado! Thanksssssss!"[1]

Now, you can buy me an avocado any day of the week, and I will express true and heartfelt gratitude to you. However, as I opened the layers of my day-to-day Life, I was unwrapping Nonsense avocado after Nonsense avocado, like a Nonsense-avocado clown car.

As much as I love avocado, I was gritting my teeth at this point and saying, "Thankssssss."

I intuited that all types of Nonsense had to stop. Not just some of the Nonsense but literally all of it. I was done. D-O-N-E in so many ways. The clown car was going to the junk yard, along with all the Nonsense avocados inside.

The late Dr. (Maya) Angelou,* in an interview with Oprah, reflected about a time when someone told a racist joke at a party she was hosting in her home. She ordered this person to leave the second she heard it. She said that nobody did that in her house, and she removed the guest.[2]

Why does that seem so radical? I wondered. But I knew why. We try so hard not to offend anyone that we literally let people run over us. That makes no sense, right? Our Lives, our energy, and our emotions are our houses, our homes. I was putting up with all sorts of crap in *my house*—real and proverbial. I was dishing out and participating in Nonsense. The combination of my texts and emails, social media interactions and friends—all of that was part of my Life too. Apparently, I had a lot of Nonsense going on in my house.

Channeling Dr. Angelou, I thought, *Nobody's gonna talk badly in my house. My Life is my house, and I don't want a house of Nonsense.*

Get out of my house, I whispered. The sensation felt strange. Powerful.

---

* Dr. Maya Angelou once said, when addressed as "Maya" by a young woman, "I'm sixty-two-years-old. I've lived so long and tried so hard that a young woman like you, or any other, has no license to come up to me and call me by my first name." Hence, I will say "Ms. Angelou" or "Dr. Angelou" here. I think it brings up an interesting debate that pairs nicely with what's coming regarding Names and Numbers. Wink wink. (*Source:* Soraya Joseph, "Maya Angelou Checks a Young Woman for Not Putting Respect on Her Name," The Grio, March 16, 2019, https://thegrio.com/2019/03/16/maya-angelou-viral.)

All the things I had made better, all the changes *had* mattered. But now I knew the magic. I knew exactly what I would be working toward. The magic? Well, the things I needed to change and eliminate now had a face and a name: NONSENSE.

When something has a face and a name, we can identify it.

We know it.

We can't unknow it.

I was looking Nonsense in the eye. I could *see* it.

Likewise, because I could see it, I knew I could do something about it.

Get out of my house.

And that's how The Year of No Nonsense began.

HOLD ON TO YOUR ASS BECAUSE HERE COMES THE RIDE

So I created a project for myself: *What if I had an entire year with no Nonsense?*

My Year of No Nonsense was epic.

I unearthed some major shit that I had been internalizing for, I don't know, all of my decades. Ugly, hard stuff—new memories, uncovered beliefs. Honestly I was sort of sorry I embarked on this little project once I was in the middle of it. During this Year, I couldn't help but think, *Stupid me. Why did I feel that I needed to get rid of Nonsense? Why was this a thing? Whose idea was this?* I wanted to run away. *What a stupid idea—a Year of No Nonsense. What freaking Nonsense this No-Nonsense Nonsense is.*

I went to the doctor because something was wrong about five months in. My whole body hurt. I was exhausted. I couldn't sleep, and when I did sleep, the sleep was never enough. Doc took blood, and a week later she called me to come into the office, giving me no explanation why. (I don't think that's ever good news, right?)

The summary: I was amazingly healthy. My bloodwork, perfect. Inflammatory markers that had plagued me for years were gone. My blood pressure was 116/75. Vitamins, minerals, thyroid, cholesterol were fine. Even my allergy sensitivities were much improved. (Thanks for the heart attack, Doc.)

So what in the world was wrong with me?

Doc looked at me and said, "I *vreally* don't know what to do with you." She is from the Middle East and incredibly blunt—which I enjoy. "You are very healthy. But you are fatter than last year. You need to eat more vegetables." *Should I be offended? Well, uh. It's true. I am fatter than last year. And I do need to eat more vegetables. Check, check.*[*]

Okay, so Doc didn't know what to do with me—her own words.

I explained to her that I was working on an experiment that acted like a daily therapy session. (I did not tell her my Year of No Nonsense idea. I was scared of what she would say, as blunt as she is.) But I said to her, "I write each morning before anyone in my house wakes up. The words fly out—some things that will never see the light of day, saved only in a folder labeled 'Do Not Use Anywhere (For Any Reason, Ever).' In summary, Doc, I begin each day with a freaking emotional and psychological bloodletting. And sometimes I freak out during and after. I am on the verge of something—and it's hard."

I shrugged.

Her eyes were big. *Did I say too much? Nah. That summed up the general logistics of this Year of No Nonsense project.* That was the project. During this time, I thought and wrote and uncovered more Truths about myself. It was a bloodletting. If I wasn't telling a personal story in my notes, I was reading methodology and psychology. I was exhausted, but motivated too.

"Okay, so you must stop *vriting* for a while," Doc said, certain that the damn writing was causing me Health problems.

"Um. No. I have to do this." I said.

"I am *vorried* about your Health. Do you need medication?" she asked.

---

[*] The Truth, as it turns out, is a big part of a Year of No Nonsense. More to come.

Oh holy night. Doc just asked me if I wanted access to her special, magical, unicorn-rainbow pharmacy. The addict in me perked up like a hound dog. I was sober—from booze—which had always been my drug of choice. (But probably only because it was the only thing I had tried.)

Oh my my. Oh hell yes. Xanax, Valium, Oxycontin, Adderall, Phentermine. Ah, phentermine! I could get high school "skinny" again! The cheater's guide to weight loss. No one would know. I could post pictures—"lowest weight in years!"—and not tell anyone that I was literally on speed.

What is wrong with you, I asked myself. I had to snap out of it, but the pharmacy—was there anything in there I needed? Maybe!

"No. No, I better not. No. No, thank you," I said nodding my head yes and saying no.

"Take care of yourself. And call me *ven* you are done with this"— waving her hands rapidly and then settling on air quotes—"'project.' You should *vee* healthier then."

Amen, sister. I thought. *A-freaking-men.*

Yes, this Year of No Nonsense "project" hurt. In the worst way.

Pretend for a minute that you have someone from another planet drop in for dinner. Your job is to explain to them what a cat is. Without using your words. Because your words are meaningless to them. That's how I felt about Nonsense. Everyone knows what a freaking cat is . . . why do I need to explain a cat?

But apparently we don't *actually* know what a cat is. Or if we do, then we aren't understanding the complexities of said cat.

The cat is a big deal.

Nonsense is a cat. A cat-avocado-clown-car. Holy shit, how in the world will I ever make sense of this . . . this, Nonsense, thing?

So my Health was okay, but everything hurt. I knew it wasn't physical. Going through this Nonsense-ridding process was an exorcism. Trying to live and articulate a Year of No Nonsense was confirmation and a subsequent attempt to release my entire Life's disappointments, Fears, Hopes, addictions, failures, trauma, and bashed Hopes. The process was a recognition and release of blame and anger. Anger and blame: two things I didn't know I hoarded so much of but also didn't realize I could also release. I did not understand the complexities of this Nonsense exorcism, because no one told me about it—well, because I started this thing. And because I started this, no one could have warned me about this squirrelly cat-not-a-cat (avocado clown car) process I patched together for myself. And finally, because I started it, I had to finish it. Cue the perfectionism tendencies. Sigh.

But growth is the theme of a well-intentioned, well-lived Life. This painful process of growth—seeking and finding Nonsense and dealing with it—is the repeatable, terrible, and necessary act that allows us to get over the past, stand strong in the present, and move toward the Life we want.

Don't be surprised if you find out more about yourself than you ever cared to know, because I know I did. Don't be surprised if the Truth, the reality stings. Maybe your body and soul will hurt like mine did.

Don't be surprised if your Life is forever changed by the Year of No Nonsense.

And if so, that won't be my doing.

That will be yours.

A GRAMMAR LESSON (OR: NONSENSE IS A PERSON, PLACE, OR THING)

A direct correlation exists between the diminishment of Nonsense and the rise of the good stuff.

For example, I have less of this Nonsense: hangovers, "frenemies," and doing races that I don't want to do. I still have some of this Nonsense: several pints of ice cream on occasion, nail biting, and gossip.

However, I don't forget or fail to take my kids to school. Likewise, the notes left on the counter for me are friendlier, less cringeworthy.

The good things continue to roll in as I have and tolerate less Nonsense. Perhaps my definition of the good things has also changed. More sleep, patience, drive (and time) to tackle projects and goals that matter to me. Presence with my family. Most simply put—I feel more alive, more purposeful and sane.

I will not tell you what in your Life is Nonsense.

Because Nonsense is mostly subjective. Mostly.

I won't tell you that exercise is the only way to get through some Nonsense. I won't say that drinking is Nonsense. You won't hear me say that ice cream is Nonsense or sitting on a couch all day knitting scarves for kitty-cats is Nonsense. One person's Nonsense is another's saving grace. Arguably, doing a triathlon is Nonsense. Perhaps writing a book about Nonsense is Nonsense.

(Summary: None of my opinions about Nonsense actually matter.)

But I am now an expert on Nonsense, if there were such a thing. I spent over two decades building my world on a foundation of Nonsense. I crafted my Life out of "I'm not good enough" materials. Made an existence contingent upon "I am a huge piece of crap" bricks and "drinking booze is my salvation" mortar. I created so much Nonsense—cities and walls of it—until I seriously had no idea what was even true or a part of me. And the crazy part was that I didn't even know Nonsense was a thing—well, until I did.

But once I knew, I could see it all.

No one can declare what Nonsense is causing you pain. Only you can identify the Nonsense in your Life. Only you can tear down (or stop building) the cities and walls that are holding you back.

Okay, so where do you start?

 Grammar is always fun, so let's begin there.

Nonsense is a noun. We all know that a noun is a person, place, or thing. Sure, Nonsense can be used to describe something ("That is nonsense!"). However, with that statement, you are also naming a person, place, or thing.

Translation: If Nonsense is a person, place, or thing, then consequently, Nonsense is *real as shit*.

You can touch it, feel it, see it, read it, and sometimes taste it or smell it. Nonsense can walk, talk, and create havoc. Nonsense can come in the form of our friends, coworkers, churchgoers, and family. Nonsense can be a place we live or work or spend our time. Nonsense can shape-shift and become a wide variety of things—from skateboarding dog videos to addiction to our very place of employment.

So, Nonsense is real but subjective.

Regardless, for the moment, let's focus on the fact that Nonsense is real, and Nonsense is also everywhere.

According to my favorite website ever, Dictionary.com, Nonsense is

1. words or language having little or no sense or meaning;
2. conduct, action, etc., that is senseless, foolish or absurd;
3. impudent, insubordinate, or otherwise objectionable behavior.[3]

Sensible definitions of Nonsense, I must say.

I went further. I found Thesaurus.com (my new favorite) and had a field day.

More synonyms for Nonsense:
babble
baloney
foolishness
madness
stupidity
trash
bananas

claptrap
hogwash
irrationality
poppycock
senselessness
thoughtlessness
And my personal favorite: rot.
But wait, I found more:
unmeaning
senseless
double-talk
buffoonery
mockery
shallowness
triviality
superficiality
trifling

Words that are not exactly synonyms but more like cousins of Nonsense were these:
gobbledygook (naturally)
lunacy
garbage
horsefeathers (huh?)
blather
swindle
fraud
flimflam
cheating[4]

Based on these definitions and synonyms, Nonsense should be easy to spot and eradicate. In theory, much of it is. I mean everyone else can spot our Nonsense a mile away, right? *Buncha busybodies.* The tough part comes when we begin to turn the mirror on ourselves. When we stop and look, openly and honestly, at ourselves, our lives, our habits, we find much more Nonsense than we probably imagined.

Research shows that our emotional skills are set by our mid-twenties and that our accompanying behaviors are, by that time, deep-seated habits.

 In other words, the stupid stuff we started doing in our twenties, we are likely to continue doing until we are in our graves.

Well, that is comforting, isn't it?

Regardless of how unsettling that is, now is the time to open our eyes. From this point forward, we must admit that we are full of Non-sense. Note: We are not Nonsense—we just have a bit of it.

If you are willing to be honest with yourself about the former (*I am full of all sorts of Nonsense*), then we are getting somewhere. If your arms are folded and your instinct is, "I do not have any Nonsense," then you are a special breed. We'll keep working.

WHY A *YEAR?*

For starters, no one knows how long it takes to change anything. Despite smart people saying it takes two weeks or twenty-one days (the most commonly touted number) or two months to change a habit, no one truly knows. According to one study, a simple, healthy habit such as exercising at lunch or eating fruit took over *sixty days* to become a habit.[5]

But we do know this: we can develop a "bad" habit in as little as two repetitions.

Gretchen Rubin, author of *The Happiness Project*, writes, "Order a doughnut with your coffee on Monday and Tuesday morning, and you'll probably find it very hard to resist ordering a doughnut on Wednesday."[6]

Let's be real: some of us just don't worry about how long it will take to create, keep, and manage all these wonderful habits. Some of us are completely unaware of our behaviors—muddling through Life, all robot-like and mad and sad. And look, I am no better than anyone else. This is Life, and it's hard.

The Year of No Nonsense is not about creating more work for yourself. You're busy. Time is short. I get it, because I was (am) the same. I had too much going on, and I was failing. I did not need another thing "to do" in my Life. I suspect you don't either. But the reality is that "too much going on" could be because 70 (80?) percent of the stuff is, you guessed it, freaking Nonsense.

The Year of No Nonsense is not about adding to your list or making space for another thing. It is about taking away, rejigging, and giving yourself room to breathe. With breath comes Life, with Life comes . . . well, Life. That's it. I like the concept of a year because it feels right. Just long enough to make real changes with enough time to mess up—a lot—and get back on track.

YOUR TYPES OF NONSENSE

I have previously provided a comprehensive (but not incredibly helpful) description of Nonsense. Words like horsefeathers, flimflam, and blather.

But we all have our Personal Brand(s) of Nonsense. Our special lies. Our horsefeathers.

That's what we need to identify: our personal horsefeathers.

For example, let's talk about Pluto. Someone decided that Pluto was no longer a planet. Who gets to decide that and why? Well, I'll tell you who: the International Astronomical Union, an organization of professional astronomers, passed two resolutions that collectively revoked Pluto's planetary status in 2006.[7] Revoked!

"I am a planet," said Pluto.

"No, you aren't."

"Aw, shit."

Poor Pluto.

Literally, the day I wrote this, I turned on CNN, and there was another group arguing that Pluto should be back in the planet game. I can't make this shit up. Then, they actually took some sort of vote a few months later—Pluto is now a "dwarf planet."[8] By the time you read this book, I wonder where Pluto will be? *Bananas*, that's where. Pluto is at the whim of someone else's words and decisions.

And that is—you guessed it—Nonsense.

So what are the types of Nonsense in your Life?

I have provided another list. And of course, this list is not comprehensive of all the potential Nonsense you're experiencing. However, if you feel like putting a check mark next to a few of these that ring your bell, then go ahead and do it.

Feel free to also add your own or cross out things you do not feel constitute Nonsense. (Pssst: It will be helpful later.)

TYPES OF NONSENSE

Self-sabotage

Blame

People pleasing

Control issues

Unworthiness

Excuses

Indecisiveness

Scarcity

Overanalysis

Self-destruction
Fear of failure
Fear of Success
Cheating
Never saying no
Never saying yes
Depression
Self-hate
Procrastination
Comparison
Perfectionism
Gossip
Addiction
Bullying
"Too busy"
Constantly seeking balance
Social media rage
Frenemies
Shame
Racism
Lying
Nutella
Keeping up with the Joneses (or Kardashians)
Stealing
Pretty much most crimes
Parenting vicariously
Hoarding
Excess
Grudges
Creating drama
Lack of accountability

Waste

Blame of self

Sexism

Living in the past

Sacrificing __ for someone else

Trying to make everyone else happy or proud

Hope mentality

Homophobia

Compulsive behaviors

Asking the wrong questions

Answering the wrong questions

Being stuck

Giving away your power

No ownership

Seeking attention

Emotional spirals

I know what you are thinking: *Every party has a pooper—that's why we invited you!* Dude, I know. This is a bummer of a list because I know that I can go through and pick out waaaaay too many of these Nonsense items in my own Life—going on right this second.

Do you see, though? Nonsense abounds. We have it everywhere. To say "I will have a Year of No Nonsense" is therefore a complete impossibility.

But do you know what is possible? And what is the point of the Year of No Nonsense?

To begin to see.

That's it. See the Nonsense. To identify it. To recognize it in a blink. Because if we can identify the Nonsense, we can then decide what to do about it. To decide "no, not today" and "never again." When we don't know that these things are horsefeathered flimflam, we cannot begin to see what's stopping so much of the good and the great from happening in our Lives.

Okay, fine, I'll get rid of Nonsense. Easy.

Ah, but some of these items have made their way into our souls, our psyches. We believe the Nonsense. We live the Nonsense. These labels, habits, attitudes, and more have infiltrated our blood, our soul, and our consciousness to the point that they have become part of us.

Therefore (attempting) to rid ourselves of Nonsense is the path to changing ourselves—big time. Ridding our Lives of (most of) the Nonsense equates to a Whole Life Overhaul. And sometimes, that's just what we need.

CHECKPOINTS AND THE YEAR OF NO NONSENSE MAP

Unfortunately (or fortunately) there is much work that surrounds the deep and powerful tentacles of Nonsense. Getting those tentacles unwrapped is not easy because, by this time in our Lives, the Nonsense is part of us. Nonsense is a warm blanket. However, we are also burning up—we like the weight of the blanket but not necessarily the heat, the pain, the itchy-scratchy.

We are busy people, and I somewhat promised that this book would not create more work for you. That's the good news. (The bad news is that I sort of lied.)

At the end of each chapter, I present you with a list of Checkpoints. And at the end of the book, you will have a Map—a Map that you create, based on your past, your present, and the Life you want—which is based on these Checkpoints. (Call 'em Rest Stops or Snack Stops or Highway Oases if you like. They are places to pause, assess, refuel.)

In other words, when you finish this book, you will have a personalized Map to guide you through your personal Year of No

Nonsense—and beyond. That is, if you work on the Checkpoints throughout.

IN PRACTICE

What is the best way to work the Checkpoints?

Answer: Whatever way you will actually do them.

From a technical standpoint, you can scribble in this book or a notebook or type in a notes app or a document. You can use the hashtags included to share on social media—to hold yourself accountable and share your journey.

If you are writing, simply create a header on your blank page: Checkpoint 1.

Then number each item under Checkpoint: 1, 2, 3.

Make your notes, exorcise the demons below each number. Checkpoint 1: 1, 2, 3.

Simple. And it will make the Mapmaking easier in the end.

The Checkpoints will not be overly burdensome, but they will necessitate some thought and action to be worth anything. And if you want a clear, easy-to-follow, and personalized Map at the end of this book, you must work through the Checkpoints.

The good news? The Checkpoints will only take a few minutes. Of course, you can spend as much time as you want.

At a minimum, read the Checkpoints—even if you refuse to write anything down. Read them. Then read them one more time, and once again. Think about the Checkpoints, just a little.

Remember: if you choose not to complete Checkpoints, you won't have your clear Map at the end. So why not just make some notes?

At a minimum, read the Checkpoints three times, and then move on.

Look, if you don't want to work, that's okay.

If you aren't ready, that's okay too.

The Checkpoints will be waiting for you. Looming. A Nonsense-reduction cloud that you can't seem to shake off. (Just kidding. Not kidding.)

· · · · Checkpoint 1 ·

1. What are two things on your Going Well List? These can be light and breezy or big Life things. But write down two things in your Life that are going well. (PS: You *do* have two. Even if all you can conjure up is breathing and this book.)

2. What are two items on your Things That Suck Ass List? Self-explanatory. What sucks right now? Do these things smell or feel like any type of Nonsense?

3. What types of Nonsense have you experienced today—you can refer to the list on page xi (Nonsense list) and pages 20–23 (Your Types of Nonsense list) to help you. Make a list of five.

4. Look again at the Nonsense lists. What do you suspect are your biggest, most frequent Nonsense offenders? What could you add or subtract?

5. Good work. First Checkpoint done. Keep going.

#YearOfNoNonsense #GoingWellList
#ThingsThatSuckAssList

2

Understanding What the Hell Happened (or Maybe Not)

*C*HILDHOOD. AH, FREAKING CHILDHOOD.*

It's easy to say, "Oh, grow up. Forget the childhood hurts and mess. You're an adult now. Act like one. Get over it. Get over yourself." Only that very statement sounds like a domineering, controlling parent, doesn't it? Children internalize criticism, and it becomes a part of who we are as adults. Telling *ourselves* to get over ourselves? Well, that takes us right back to the root of some real mess—criticism, contempt, and other Nonsense.[1] *Stand up straight. Mind your manners. Don't talk back. Stop biting your nails. Lose that attitude. Don't sass me. What I did TO you isn't a big deal NOW. Move on.*

We must look at the Nonsense that may be our childhood. And begin to unravel how the Nonsense of our childhood may have

---

* As an initial matter, I am not a therapist or medical professional. You know that by now. While I dive into some "heavy" topics and provide my own anecdotes and personal spin, it's important to know my place in this world—I do—and your unique Life and mental Health are not my expertise. Only you are the expert of yourself, and please remember to seek professional care and medical advice when your Health is involved.

unraveled us. On the bright side, we humans have the innate capacity
to self-heal. We need not continue reliving or being stuck in the past
or in the wrongs of our childhood—we can move forward. We can
thrive. We can Live.

But first, we need to *see*.*

Look, I grew up "privileged," but that's a wide-swinging term
that has many dimensions, from status to race to able-bodied. People
get upset talking about it—and understandably. For my intent and
purpose, I want to point out that privileged is not a synonym for
nurtured; it is not a synonym for a trauma-free childhood, unicorns
and freaking rainbows. I want to caution against assumptions about
privilege—it's a complex topic.[2]

I won't defend my suffering, and you shouldn't defend yours.
No one knows and understands what someone else's childhood was
like. One facet might appear as privilege, but it might be something
else, too. What might look like poverty might be nurturing, love, and
support. We did not choose to be born, or in the bodies we have. We
did not choose our parents, our childhoods, our schools, our bodies,
our environments. It is important to not compare and assume. That's
called being a good human. (More on this in Chapter 6.)

Before we dig into the likely unraveling caused by growing up, I
want to bring up a concept that has proved helpful when thinking of
childhood.† The fact that Life is allowed to be a paradox. It means that
something doesn't have to be all one thing—our childhoods don't
have to be all bad, our jobs not completely 100 percent terrible, our
spouses not total idiots, and our lives not fully and totally shit. We
can have good and bad, short and tall, big and small. We can have a

---

* You will get tired of reading how important it is to "see." There's a reason for repeti-
tion. Because seeing is the most important component of the Year of No Nonsense.

† I found reading about the Enneagram super helpful when beginning to unravel my
own childhood. A great resource is *The Wisdom of the Enneagram: The Complete Guide to Psychological and Spiritual Growth for the Nine Personality Types* by Don Richard Riso and Russ Hudson.

mess, and we can also heal from said mess. Dr. Seuss had it right, with all his paradoxically true word books.

But this recognition about paradox triggered a massive break-through for me. Maybe this is not news to you. Perhaps you are accustomed to the great nature of the world: good and evil, yin and yang. But the application for me was helpful: I am permitted to be not-so-thrilled about parts of my past, but I am also allowed to be grateful for the lessons the past taught me. I can recognize that many important emotional needs may not have been met, but I gained Grit, resilience, and creativity. I can understand some trauma and how that has impacted me and also see a path to move forward. People have hurt me, but those same people supported me, loved me, and never intended to impart pain, even though they did.

Paradox is a very helpful tool for me, which is why I mention it here. We are not required to be black-and-white about our lives—we can be all the colors of the rainbow and every shade in between.

So childhood.

A young woman with a higher ACE score* is "four and half times as likely to become depressed and is twelve times as likely to take her own Life."[3] Experiences during childhood matter, and their impact may result in an adult crisis that has been swept under the rug.

During my Year of No Nonsense, I learned that seeing *what is* and *what was* is a fundamental requirement for change. In seeing, I uncovered some dysfunction and pain about my past—that has impacted my present. In seeing, I opened up floodgates of emotion, because the things I uncovered have direct correlations to the biggest types of Nonsense I struggle with: self-esteem, addiction, anxiety, Fear, intimacy issues, toxic Core Beliefs—to name a few.

---

* An ACE score is a tally of different types of abuse (physical or emotional), neglect, and other hallmarks of a rough childhood. According to the Adverse Childhood Experiences study, the more brutal your childhood, the higher your score is likely to be and the higher your risk for later Health problems.

My recent uncoverings made me mad, yes. I was grateful for this though, the unveiling of the core of my Truth—as some call it in psychology—the primal wound.[4] In learning my primal wound, I was able to understand and explain so much of my pain and suffering and show compassion to myself. After all this pain, addiction, and suffering?[5] What did I learn? I learned and proved to myself that I wasn't crazy. I wasn't broken. And I could change and heal. I just had a wound that needed to be triaged, dealt with—and then I needed to handle the remaining aftershock injuries.

I paused long and hard about stories I included in this book, knowing that I was taking an emotional risk—on many levels—with myself, my family, with readers. After all, this book is about breaking through Nonsense, not reliving past wrongs, blaming, or being a stuck record, skipping and replaying the same childhood garbage sound, over and over again.

In the eleventh hour, I cut out many of the specific stories about my childhood. But many remain.

The last thing I want to be is another author acting like she had a hard Life. But here's the thing: I did have a hard childhood. And it's very likely that—if you picked up this book—you did too.

This book is not pretending that I grew up on the streets, didn't have food to eat or a roof over my head. I am white and able-bodied. I was never homeless. Yes, people have had and will have it way worse. But comparison of suffering is toxic (Chapter 5). I did encounter violence and abuse, Fear and terror, shame and uncertainty, some of it in the name of religion and God. I have an unreasonably high ACE score for someone so "privileged." I tried to end my Life once and thought about it probably thousands of times, starting from age six. One of my earliest suicidal thoughts was in first grade—when I cut my hair short—and a classmate called me a fat boy and I swear I felt my family shirk away from me, too. I was seven years old. I fought a battle with booze for almost twenty years—a battle that almost claimed my Life time and time again. I have no shame in any of this, but I also know that my wounds are not hollow or "privileged." Neither are yours.

As a parent myself, I am in a constant state of Fear that I am causing irreparable damage to my children—making their childhoods a weave of mess they will have to later unravel. After all, parenting is a skill—we all begin without any real tools or actual skillset.

Where we fail as parents? Thinking we know everything and there is nothing to learn; assuming our parents got it all right and repeating their same patterns; thinking that we own our children and exist to control them (more on this later). So I continue to ask myself, *Am I saying the wrong things? Am I doing the wrong things? How do I know this is best for them? How do I put my own ego aside to ensure these kids Live their best Lives?*

When I think about my childhood—as a parent of a tween boy and girl—I find myself stumped about many of my experiences and feelings. I believe my parents did the best they knew in raising me. I am trying to believe the same about all people (that they are doing the best that they can). In Chapter 6, I talk about why I believe this to be true (Dr. Brené Brown). I also lean heavily on the quote "When you know better, you do better" (Dr. Maya Angelou). Where I struggle is when there is clearly no desire on the part of the Other People to know or do better.

"Many of the expectations we have of our children are unspoken. Despite what we don't put into words, children intuitively sense when we wish them to be other than they are . . . that we want them to fulfill our fantasies of who they will grow up to be, and what they will accomplish. Yes, some children rise to this challenge and are successful. But for every child who does there are a host of others who buckle under the pressure."[6]

And what does "buckling under pressure" look like? *Addiction. Disordered eating. Personality disorders. Anxiety. Depression. Sexual dysfunction.* To name a few.

This book isn't about blame, though. It's about Nonsense.

But blame, if used incorrectly, is a form of Nonsense.

My memories of childhood were not good, which simply made me feel like an ungrateful brat as an adult. It wasn't until recently that I realized that my memories were real, my suffering valid, and the sadness erupted from a place of Truth. *When you know better, you simply do better. People pleasing runs deep and dark.*

Again, this is a book about Nonsense. I write these things because I am not the same person I was ten years ago or ten minutes ago— and it never occurred to me that all of my suffering had a reason and origin. Not fault, not a place to point fingers—but a birthplace. Then Nonsense perpetuated it all.

"You are not crazy."[7]

I hope that by talking about my struggles, pain, and experiences, you might see some of yourself—and then you can be on the road to your best Life. I write this book, because in the last few years I realized how common Nonsense is. And to get where I am now—on the path to healing—I had to start where I was. I had to look at my past. I had to *see.*

I had to find the primal wound, triage it, and stop the bleed.

To move forward, *you may* have to do the same.

You may need to look back a little, you have to *see.* You don't have to revisit your childhood or even know what happened—only that something did. So understanding what the hell happened? That might just be impossible, destructive, or less than desirable.[8] You may find some of yourself in my story or you may be repulsed by the things I write. Either way is fine with me, because this is my Truth (more on this later).

Becoming a parent catapulted me into this painful exploration of learning how to parent. To really learn, I had to look at my experiences as a child. It was an exploration that I could no longer shove onto the back burner—because it was starting to boil over in other ways, and I was drowning in the hot water.

* * *

When my daughter, Stella, was nine years old, I took her to Madison, Wisconsin, for the CrossFit Games, a massive event over several days. At the Games, "The Fittest on Earth" take on about a dozen events featuring endurance, strength, agility, flexibility, and speed. The Games are grueling and fun to spectate—from the food to the fit bodies everywhere.

Stella is strong and moves her body freely. At her age, I was terrified of my changing body. I was scared that I took up too much space. I felt that I couldn't move in a way that was acceptable for sport or, hell, Life in general. When I saw that she willingly chose a sports bra and booty shorts as an outfit and loved to do burpee challenges, I figured the Games would be a killer event for her.

Translation: I was eagerly awaiting my "Mom of the Year" award when we returned.

I didn't know how well an almost-ten-year-old would do at an event that lasted literally from morning until evening—for damn near a week. It was definitely a parenting gamble. But she was amazing, and we had a great time—for the first three days.

On the fourth day everything changed.

The cherub child turned into a moody teenager. One second we were holding hands in the coliseum. The next minute, she said, "Don't talk to me."

In that moment, even though I was quite annoyed, I thought about what the human—that child of mine—was trying to prove with *don't talk to me*. Thankfully, I had been reading Dr. Shefali Tsabary and her words of "conscious parenting." She urges parents to accept that a child is a divine spirit, a person who has their own feelings, ideals, and ways of thinking. That they are another human—one not to be owned or controlled.[9] Even though they are not grown humans. (I am ashamed to say that was revolutionary thinking for me.)

"Love without consciousness becomes need, dependency; it becomes control in the name of love. That's what we are doing with our children."
—DR. SHEFALI TSABARY[10]

Stella had gotten a tad snotty that morning. She wanted to wear the same shirt from the first day—it was stinky. I decided to accept the situation and let her wear the stinky shirt. Something that would have never happened for me as a child, as my mom and I went into fight-to-the-death battle over this type of thing. I realized, though, that Stella's stinky shirt did not matter. And really, it was her choice. What did I care? Honestly. We compromised on the shorts though—but not in a domineering way. I just reasoned with her, *Look, you can wear a stinky shirt, but you can't wear stinky shorts, because that's unsanitary and here's why.* Made sense to her. *Little human.* She bought that argument, and we reached an agreement.

My friend Susan has raised five (!) daughters, and I often ask her advice about parenting. Over text, she had implored me not to allow Stella's attitude at the Games to affect me—no matter what she said or did during the week, to continue to be me. Not to tolerate disrespect, but not to get emotional about it. Susan wrote, "Act like everything is the best and you are super excited. Don't let her know that her attitude is affecting you."

So on the fourth day when Stella said, "Don't talk to me," I was prepared. I put myself in Stella's place. I recognized that I get crabby for no reason too. Why was Stella not entitled to feel the same way?

Susan said that she will tell her daughters, "If you want to be in a crappy mood, fine. But go do it over there, because I don't want to be around it. I will give you some space, but you will not be disrespectful to me."

I had an idea. I grabbed my bag, and I told Stella, "I'll be back."

Her eyes got big. "Where are you going?" she asked.

"I'm just going to step out for a minute and give you some space. I'll be right up there," I said, pointing to the coliseum section entry.

Before she could respond, I was gone. I stayed away about ten minutes, pretending that I was on the phone or whatnot, with her in my line of sight (of course). She would glance up at me every so often.

When I returned, I cheered and acted excited. In no time, she got right back on board.

On the way to the hotel that night, I simply asked her, "Why were you mad at me? When you asked me not to talk to you?"

She said, "I just needed you to be quiet. I don't know why."

I said, "I understand. Sometimes I get pissy too."

Parenting tip: use of the word "pissy" sends any kid into fits of giggles. And that was how the day ended: with laughter (and pizza).

Stella and I have managed a new level of communication and comaraderie since that trip. I pray that it lasts, but more than that? I am *conscious* of our relationship; I will do whatever it takes to maintain it; I *see* it. I constantly remind myself that she is a person and a divine spirit, just as she is. *Tiny human.*

That, like me, she has bad days and is entitled to feel certain ways and to express those feelings. Any childhood trauma is exacerbated by parents suppressing our feelings or invalidating our sense of self by pumping up theirs. My role as a parent is to guide, to help her expressions in the realm of appropriateness—not to own and overpower—to be a part of her Life, not the puppeteer of it. (I do the same with my son, by the way.)

My job (as a parent) is to be a support for my children. The children are not here to fulfill my needs. They are not here for me to burden with emotional baggage from my Life. They are not here to reflect my own "greatness" (or lack thereof). I am here to support them in their journey of growing up—not dictate how their journey goes. We are here to open doors; it is the child's choice whether to walk through them.[11]

Kind and proper discipline is an act of love and support.* We want children to become the best version of themselves—not feral children devoid of Life skills and incapable of contribution. The problem is: most of us haven't grown up ourselves, so we are "teaching" and "raising" when we have not dealt with our own "lack."[12] Children are not here to make up for our mistakes, to fulfill our missed opportunities, or to become our points of blame.

 All of the foregoing is to say—maybe you are a parent or maybe not, but you **were** a child. And childhood matters.

Just imagine if we all had been treated as "divine beings" and entitled to have emotions and opinions growing up. What if we were disciplined appropriately and without rage or anger? What if there was no emotional or sexual abuse, inappropriate behavior and ickiness, secrets and tickling gone way too far? What would our lives have looked

---

* "Even the most assiduous of parents cannot fully protect their children, even if they lock them in the basement, safely away from drugs, alcohol, and internet porn. In that extreme case, the too-cautious, too-caring parent merely substitutes him- or herself for the other terrible problems of life. This is the great Freudian Oedipal nightmare. It is far better to render Beings in your care competent than to protect them. . . . Question for parents: do you want to make your children safe, or strong?" (Jordan B. Peterson, 12 *Rules for Life* [New York: Random House Canada, 2018], 47). Dr. Shefali Tsabary might perhaps argue that we don't make our kids either, but the impact of unconscious parenting has an impact.

like? Some of us were treated and raised in a positive, safe space. But I would be willing to bet that the bigger-than-believable majority of us were raised in a place that felt or was, in fact, unsafe. Or raised as mini versions of our parents, made in their image, expected to be perfect, and expected to do as they said. Not as divine beings with feelings, minds, and hearts of our own. Or perhaps children were to be seen and not heard. What if we had been heard? What if we had been allowed to be heard? What if someone had wanted to actually hear what we had to say?

Childhood is often the great obstacle that we must overcome. Many of us are clinging to the past and blaming childhood for our adult mistakes, tendencies, and myriad ways of being stuck. And perhaps rightly so. It very well might be to blame.

Most Core Beliefs we hold are straight outta childhood.[13] If we don't recognize where they come from, we can't do a damn thing about course correcting ourselves as adults—when we must grow up and be who we are meant to be. I suffered through years of addiction to deal with some of these Core Beliefs. I drank so I didn't have to face any of the hurts, disappointments, and pains of my past. I knew something was wrong, but I didn't know what—so I dove into the darkness of alcohol and self-loathing—where I could be invisible. *I am not good enough. I will never be fit. I will never have enough. Scarcity. Imperfection. Hard to love.*

Look, I am terrified of the imperfect things I am imparting to my kids. My oldest, James, will likely write a book about the ways I screwed up his Life. He frequently says, "Stop yelling, Mom" and "Why are you so 'yelly'?" (And I swear, I'm not even raising my voice.) But during those times, I am speaking in a disappointed or aggravated tone and he hears yelling. He hears my disappointment. Then I am angry at myself for doing that to him—it feels too familiar, and I freak out.

So my main parenting goal? Try to be less "yelly."

Trauma may be an underestimated part of our past as well.[14] But I don't have trauma, we might think. But trauma's working definition can be "anything that is too much, too soon, or too fast for our nervous system to handle, especially if we can't reach a successful resolution."[15] Trauma can be low humming—something that makes a low buzzing sound in the background for far too long. We hear the buzz but have no idea what that sound is. We just know it is flipping us out—which results in real issues and how we process things as adults.

Exploring past trauma is not fun and, of course, is outside the scope of this book (and should only be ventured into with professional help). But trauma may be a real part of our past and, subsequently, our present. Worse, we had no idea, because we have pushed down the experiences of our childhood. All we know is that we feel scared, ashamed, addicted, and full of Nonsense. Chances are, if those emotions are bubbling up, there is something unresolved—and we may need to accept that something is there before we can move past it.

Childhood matters.

We don't need to dredge up the list of painful experiences either. But we may need to acknowledge that something happened—and it mattered.[16] As I moved from child to teenager, I stepped into feelings, trauma, and issues from young childhood. And some of these things I turned into Core Beliefs. They became beliefs whether such things were true or not. So I look at my kids and I think, *What Core Beliefs am I putting into them or reinforcing? Are those good things or destructive? What are they experiencing that is "too much, too soon, or too fast" and how can I help? (So help me God.)*

As an adult with a heavy lean toward disordered eating and addiction, I realized I had unknowingly absorbed destructive beliefs from childhood. The beliefs hurt, and I subconsciously wanted to suppress them. I wanted to not feel. I wanted numbness. As I transitioned out of addiction and began to identify Nonsense in my Life,

I was able to see these beliefs for what they were and how they mattered. Not in a blame way but in a way to get past what was hurting me in the present, in the now.

I saw the identification of the trauma and pain (and Nonsense) of the past as a way to heal, to change, to set boundaries, and to move on.

Translation: we need to recognize our past pain and clean up our Nonsense to heal, yes. We need to do it for ourselves. But also, we need to do it so we don't dump these burdens on our children, students, and the next generation in our Lives.

MOVING PAST SHAME: GET OUT OF YOUR OWN WAY

Blaming others is a surefire route to get the onus off oneself—to divert responsibility.

But it's also useless and ineffective. Sure, we can blame effectively, but for the most part, we must take responsibility for all the things in our corner. Our corners, however, may look like a quite damning episode of Emotional *Hoarders* also.

Regardless, there is a vast difference between responsibility and awareness, acceptance and mere understanding of what happened. Some parts are not our fault—at all—and we need not take responsibility for those things.

Understanding what happened to you (or because of you)—or simply that something happened and you don't know what—can quickly trigger shame. Embarrassment about who you are, where you came from, what you did or didn't do, what you caused or thought you caused, and what was done (or not done) to you, for you.

The list of shame might be longer than the list of Nonsense.

So what about shame? Shame often runs deep; it is dark and hidden. Lovely synonyms for shame? *Blot. Self-disgust. Pang.* Yes. Yes. Yes.

Shame:

the painful feeling arising from the consciousness
of something dishonorable, improper, ridiculous,
etc., done by oneself or another[17]

My biggest source of shame is—and has always been—around
my body. The whole body—every inch of it—is a vessel of shame.

When I was a child, someone pointed out that my nipples were
"weird" because they didn't stick out. I may have been seven years
old—about the same time I cut my hair short. (It was a good year.)
I didn't know what that meant, about weird nipples, until someone
gave those weird nipples a name: *inverted*. Because I was a nerd, I went
to the dictionary and looked up the word "inverted."

"Turned upside down." *My nipples are turned upside down?? No freaking
wonder everyone is staring at me. I'm headed straight for the Barnum and Bailey.*

And thus began the slow decline of my tits.

Needless to say, I was not a teenage girl to show off my boobs.
Inverted. Then I heard someone say that large nipples were "gross,"
which made me question, *Oh man! Are mine large? Small? How would I know?
What does the dictionary say?* (Nothing on this.)

I wore a hot pink two-piece bathing suit when I was sixteen. It
was my first summer of wearing bikinis, and I felt good in it. Until
an older boy from church let me know that he could see my nipples through it—*Inverted! Oh God!*—and that he wished I would put
on a T-shirt because it gave him dirty thoughts. *Shame. Please forgive
me, God.*

Shortly after, I got into trouble for making out with my perfectly
nice, sweet boyfriend in the yard. Shamed, made to feel like trash—a
slut—even though I was just kissing a boy. A nice boy, who I really,
really liked. *Whore.* I was told by another friend's mother that I was

a bad influence, and I had to leave a party. *Trash.* I was at a party my senior year, and a guy friend of mine started kissing me. He put his hand under my shirt and asked me what was wrong with my nipples, and "Where *are* they?" *Shame. Again.*

So you might wonder what is actually wrong with my boobs. *Abso-freaking-nothing.* I am happy to report that the *near-fatal inversion flaw* took care of itself. My set looks and acts like any other non-surgically-enhanced, post-two-baby pair in any random locker room in the country. They are fine—and I'll say, hell, even better than fine.

But I never knew that.

Because by the time I was seventeen years old, I had no less than half a dozen people comment on my tits—discuss them, point out whatever—which humiliated me beyond Life, space, and time. *Weird. Shame. Cover yourself. Dirty thoughts.* The memory remained long, long after the action.

Shame. Body shame. I am shameful.

The shame extended to the rest of my body, to my hips, my ass, my weight. It extended to sexuality. The shame extended to other parts of my body—like a small birthmark on my stomach, a pattern of freckles on my shoulder.

My body was a place of Fear for me. And not a damn ounce of it was my fault. There was the dermatologist (yes, really) who touched my vagina and said, "She's going to start puberty soon." (I'm not sure that's necessary—you know—to diagnose a kid with "puberty," especially as a skin doc.) The youth leader at camp who stared at me and licked his lips each time he saw me. The older men who brushed up against me, the ones who drove by my house, slowly—over and over again. People who should not have dumped their secrets and stories on me. Those who should not have touched me—ever—and especially not while talking to me about "important things" or "Godly things." Those who continued to touch, grab, or pinch me when I pulled away—time and time again—asserting their power and place over my own fucking body without my consent or care. *This is not okay!* These are the stories that so many of us have. *Fear. Slut. Not Good Enough. Come back here! Where are you going? It's just a hug.*

By the time I had a new marriage under my belt, my body was not, in fact, a wonderland—it was a wasteland.

A wasteland that had been lit on fire and burned for nearly two decades. *Shame.* I didn't want anyone to look at it. God forbid anyone touch me—I couldn't stand it. I had to get blasted to have sex. The mild exception was my husband, who I didn't want to look at me either—touch (when drunk) but don't look, please. *Lights off, buster!* After plunging into law school and never once recognizing the shame I was carrying around, I began to treat my body like the worst part of me. Because, well, I thought it was.

I drank uncontrollably. I ate so much, all the time, and food that was garbage. I do remember a period when I had to think about the last time I had eaten something green. *Two weeks? A month?*

I just wanted my body to explode, I think. I ballooned up to over 250 pounds. This was before children, mind you. I had all the time in the world to work on myself—to work out, eat well, bask in the freaking sun and glory of my twenties. Instead, I hid in a dark room. I wrote. I drank. I downloaded music, and I sank into a place from which I wasn't sure I would ever emerge. I didn't want to emerge. I just wanted to forget I existed.

The darkness consumed me long after I recovered from a dark plunge (more on this later).

After marriage—even though I can report I was saved by marriage, by some sense of freedom—the darkness still continued. Long after law school. Even after children came. I had moments of joy and Happiness but many waves of darkness. I carried tremendous shame about my body despite losing some weight, wearing heels and suits to court, and even starting to swim, bike, and run. I carried shame around being a mom and the way I didn't know if I loved my children enough or cared for them like I should.

I was no longer on such an obvious path of mad destruction, but I was on the slow-burn decline. I suppose I was on a socially acceptable path to dying: one sad, shameful, slow, alcohol-infused day at a time.

I can (now) trace all of this darkness directly to the shame I felt around my body and trauma from my past. (Which is why we stay in our heads only—so we don't have to feel our bodies.)[18]

That was not my fault—I didn't know that my body was okay, safe, and secure. Because my world didn't feel safe. No one actually confirmed that I was safe. In fact, quite the opposite—I was raised to Fear. Fear was used as a weapon for love and control. God was to be feared. Parents feared. Failure, kidnapping, hurricanes, regrets, and dogs: Fear. I did not intuit I was safe, because, well . . . I wasn't.

And forget being safe in my body. It's not like you can look to the media to tell you that you are safe and your body is okay if home isn't delivering. My body was better than fine, actually—beautiful. It wasn't until I started triathlon that I learned my body was a bloody freaking miracle. I actually birthed and fed two children (with my inverted-not-inverted nipples, mind you) in some giant feat of the miracle of Life, and it took the sport of triathlon to inform me that my body was "okay."

I can count my blessings in the realm of massive self-improvement, because I am "okay" today. When I look back at these stories, I know that I am good even. I can't deny how far I have come in this journey—this clearing of the thorny path to self-acceptance. This space of being a survivor—a word I only recently aligned myself with. The path was not instant; it was a journey. I've been beaten, worn, and pained by said journey.

Now I wear a swimsuit the second the weather warms up—even a little sooner. Why? Because I utterly wasted my twenties and most of my thirties thinking I had a wasteland for a body. I'm not wasting another day of my body—whatever it looks like. I am trying desperately to Live in the body I have—not outside of it—but in it. For myself, sure. But also because I have two children—a boy and a girl—who look to me for cues about not only body image but also safety and emotional stability.

I want to show them both that I'm not ashamed of living in my body, that it's safe to be in your body (even though it is sometimes only by the grace of God that I can even walk out on the pool deck wearing anything but a trash bag). It's important for me to stand out there strong and (mostly) proud in the skin I am in. It's not just about me. I can do it for my kids and others at the pool who might need to see that strong, athletic, and proud comes in many sizes. (Even if inside I don't feel all those things all the time.) That maybe even if I am a real-time "before" picture, I am also—not.

I put on a tiny bikini on a recent family trip. The thing was truly small and made of strings. I don't know what I was trying to prove. Perhaps because I wore sweaters in summer for so long, I have reacted in a completely opposite way.

Regardless, my eleven-year-old son said, "My gosh, Mom!" And put his hands over his eyes.

Automatically, I assumed that it was because he thought I was too jiggly to wear it out.

I said, "Son, I have worked my tail off for this body! I am showing it off. No matter what it looks like."

He said, "That's great, Mom. I know. But that bathing suit is made of string. What happens if it comes untied? What happens then?" his eyes wide.

Always the practical one. He wasn't even paying any mind to my body. He was concerned that my bathing suit was held together by string.

You may feel like the struggle with not loving (but wanting to love) your body will always exist. (Lawd knows I wonder.)

But doing the work to uncover where that body shame *started* empowers you to look that shame right in the eyes. Once you see the source of the shame, you can begin to change it. When you change it—you make space to feel worthy of that glorious warm sun on your skin . . . completely and unapologetically. (Slathered with sunscreen, of course.)

OH HEY, HI! SELF-AWARENESS

But. Discovering what causes us shame and looking that shame in the eye requires a certain amount of self-awareness.

Self-awareness is the ability to assess oneself realistically. To see what is true about ourselves.[19]

Not all of us are born with this little gem; we all have that friend who is completely self-unaware. Unfortunately, sometimes we are that friend. But self-awareness is an important tool in the Nonsense-ridding arsenal.

Self-awareness is a bitch. Because in order to be authentic and self-aware, we must know (and sometimes accept) the tough Truth about ourselves and perhaps the bullshit that we are selling to ourselves and others. Then we must be equipped to imagine (then carve) a path through Life that navigates these things. Not dramatically, not negatively—simply realistically. In other words, you *have* fat—you *are* not fat. You have *anger*—you are not an *angry person*. How you frame yourself is part of self-awareness. Looking at your characteristics and habits from an objective, almost scientific angle is key to true self-awareness.

Many times we are unable to see the good in ourselves, but we also refuse to see the sticking points, the "bad" habits, and the issues that we must address—not to be perfect but to lead the Lives we are meant to Live.

Some of the most self-aware people are the happiest because they possess a thing called Emotional Intelligence. And one thing is certain in this world: Emotional Intelligence increases with age.[20]

Emotional Intelligence is not something that we are born with. "Emotional intelligence is born largely in the neurotransmitters of the brain's limbic system, which governs feelings, impulses and drives. Research indicates that the limbic system learns best through motivation, extended practice, and feedback."[21]

In other words, we must work to not be an emotional mess, to not be a disaster in Life and relationships. We must strive to not kill ourselves or others. We are not wired for Happiness—quite the opposite (more on this later). In other words, rarely are people not working against the disaster that is simply the act of doing Life. As Jordan B. Peterson puts it, "Life is suffering. That is clear."[22] If Life is tough—and barreling toward us—then of course, "Building one's emotional intelligence cannot—will not—happen without sincere desire and concerted effort."[23]

Dang it. Nothing is easy, is it? In a way—but our suffering is part of our mind, our expectations (also more on this later).

So in essence, a self-aware individual understands his or her values, goals, desires, wants—and bullshit. Someone who lacks self-awareness finds it easy to make decisions that "bring on inner turmoil by treading on buried values."[24] Buried values?

Treading on buried values sounds like a fancy way of saying living a Life that is not authentically yours. Treading on buried values sounds like a gut punch. Sounds also a lot like suffering—because that's exactly what it is.

CORE BELIEFS

If, several years ago, someone had asked me what my Core Beliefs or values were, I would have regurgitated something like, "I believe in God. Family is important. Life should be full of Happiness. Butterflies and rainbows would be bitchin' also." You know, the things you are supposed to say if you Live on the planet and want to be a "Good Girl."*

So what are Core Beliefs?

To greatly simplify this process, here's the quick and dirty. We all have certain "Core Truths," which consist of a repetitive pattern of behaviors and thoughts that are shaped by our internal expectations and our assumptions about ourselves and the world—and these are collected as "Truths" over the course of our Lives (think: childhood). We therefore feel and experience day-to-day Life through these conventions, expectations, and ideas.

Subsequently, we manufacture "belief systems—our Core *Beliefs*" out of these collected truths. Then our Core Beliefs cause us "to develop *Active* Beliefs—how we operate in the world." These so-called Active Beliefs then support outcomes that back up and support our Core Beliefs. "The whole system is a giant double feedback loop, each element both encompassing and contained within the other."[25]

If someone pressed me further a few years ago about my real Core Beliefs—like maybe after I had a few drinks and my guard was down—I might have told more Truth:

"I believe that I will always be overweight, slow, sad, and somewhat miserable." Or maybe "I will never get out of debt." Or maybe "I am not worthy of love, so get the hell away from me and stop trying to love me. I am hard to love." Ah-hem.

Core Beliefs are windows into our behaviors and the reasons we do the things we do—good and bad and everywhere in between. Simply: the things we hold as true.[26]

---

* By the way, can we all pause for a minute and promise ourselves, the world, and the Universe *never* to use the term "Good Girl" again? Thanks.

Sometimes we might not even know we hold these beliefs, but something as modest as an encounter with a certain type of person will reveal them. Think about how you react when you see a homeless person on the street. Is your first reaction to empathize—to think, *That could be me*—and give them assistance in whatever form you can? Or is the first reaction to think, *They should get their shit together*? Or (perhaps even worse) do you just pretend they don't exist?

Turns out what we think about someone else says way more about us than we might have thought—or are willing to admit. In *Blink*, Malcolm Gladwell analyzes the first impression and where it comes from. While many explanations such as upbringing, status, and racial bias all weigh into our first impressions, Core Beliefs also drive "blink" impressions, "gut" reactions and instincts.

I was hauling around some pretty tragic Core Beliefs. I had no idea that some of my thoughts about myself, marriage, and Life were so dark and so deeply ingrained inside me. Basically, I was operating my ship based off them.

1. I will never be fit or healthy.
2. Marriage is a prison.
3. Money will always be a struggle.
4. Careers are not meant to be fulfilling.

And the big one:

5. I am hard to love.

HARD TO LOVE

Before I got married, my dad told my now husband, "Good luck, son. She is hard to love."

He was trying to be funny—an exclamation point on his approval granting my delicate Southern hand in marriage. I also think that my dad would be the last person in the world to intentionally hurt me.

But intent does not negate impact, and sometimes the people who "love" us the most leave the biggest wounds.[27]

I know, too, that when people are joking, they are telling some version of *their* Truth—or perhaps fulfilling some need by the words. Maybe it's not *your* Truth. But it's someone's Truth.

It wasn't until the Year of No Nonsense that I realized how much that statement had impacted me. A statement made by a man who had loved me so much and controlled me so tightly that his Truth unintentionally harmed me. His Truth was that he probably didn't want me to ever leave home or get married, to grow up, to be independent of him—despite the lip service he gave me about independence. He projected that I was hard to love to hide his own pain of me flying away. He needed me to need him. That's my interpretation as he and I continue to work through our relationship. I had, however, tucked that one away—into my Core Beliefs. I am not sure how my husband moved forward after being told this little gem about his soon-to-be wife. But I went into my marriage thinking, *This marriage thing will be tricky. Especially since I am hard to love.*

Only marriage didn't feel that hard—until I upped the ante on my body-image issues and cultivated a more serious drinking problem— all stemming from the same childhood bullshit wounds. *My body is gross. I am hard to love. Marriage doesn't feel that hard. Maybe I should do something to make it harder . . . since I am hard to love and my body is disgusting. I should make myself hard to love. To live up to the Truth of the fact that I am hard to love and proving the fact that my body is shameful.*

A few years back, I gave a small-group talk where I discussed the "marriage is a prison" Core Belief of mine: when I was angry, upset, or something about marriage fluffed me up, my go-to reaction was, "PRISON! Get me out of this marriage prison. I'm trapped." The group was mostly moms, with kids ranging from babies to teenagers, from all walks of Life. I was coming off the Year That Could Kiss My Ass, so I was a little worn.

I have done some big work breaking apart that particular Core Belief. Understanding that now, a committed relationship is meant to be a partnership—not a prison. After all, I left a childhood of Black Hawk control and jumped right into a marriage. I had no freedom or feeling of safety for so long, and I didn't fight for any—because I didn't know that I needed to. Naturally, when I got married, it was easy to transition to marriage as a prison.

I relayed this Core Belief to the crowd of women. About half were scribbling in their notebooks, the other half were staring holes through my head, and one was on her phone playing Candy Crush (there's always one, for the love). *Well, this is unsettling.*

I took a breath. Apparently, this group of unicorns all had great relationships and none felt imprisoned. Duly noted. Okay, so on to parenting. . . .

"*Motherhood* is a prison," I said.

Everyone, even Candy Crush, popped their heads up. There was a rustle and then silence. I had hit the right nerve.

"Right?" I said. "Is there a greater prison than parenting?"

The moms stared, but they were listening.

I continued, "Regardless of how precious our children are. Regardless of how much we love them—motherhood is a total trap. Once you enter the World of Mom, you are in it. You can be willingly pinned beneath a sleeping toddler. You can be trapped at soccer practice, at carpool. You are trapped into making lunches and baths and school supply shopping. You are trapped within teenage attitudes, cell phones, groundings, homework, debates, fights, and struggles. Parenting is an absolute place of no return. Even if you *lose* a child, God forbid, you are trapped in that hell of grief for Life. All things children, all a prison."

I waited for them to walk out, but no one left.

I looked at the small group. "This is precisely the whole idea of Core Beliefs. Whatever we believe in our hearts and souls, we will embody. We will operate with that set of principles in mind. We will go forth believing and acting this way."

At that moment, I asked the group to write down some of their negative Core Beliefs on pieces of paper and pass them to me.

I read out loud from scraps of paper they turned in. The list was unsettling.

It was also hauntingly familiar.

I am disgusting.

I am alone.

No one loves me.

No one will love me.

I am worthless.

I am unimportant.

I am stupid.

I am a terrible mother.

I am crazy.

I am invisible.

I am weak.

I am slow.

I will die alone.

In other words, some amazing people are carrying around some tough Core Beliefs—many of which are lies we have been told or are telling ourselves—and adopted as Truth.[28] Here's the kicker: whether they are objectively true or not matters nil, because in our hearts, they are Truth.

Some of these Core Beliefs are absolutely horsefeathered Nonsense. For now, we just need to find what beliefs are there: good, bad, right, wrong, true, or false, we need to get to the place where we have identified these beliefs. Maybe it doesn't matter how the beliefs arrived; but we need to make sure we see them. (Unfortunately, naming our Core Beliefs sometimes tells us where they come from. *Ah-hem, there it is again—childhood.* I'm sorry.)

Maybe you see some of your Core Beliefs in the list. Maybe not. But you do have some Core Beliefs. We all do. And maybe it requires some digging. This book is your shovel. Keep digging.

NEVER ENOUGH

Growing up, I wanted to write—articles or books—didn't matter. I simply wanted to write. I could see *who I was to become* with every fiber of my being from a young age—and it was not an attorney.

I was perhaps to become a journalist. I felt like I would be a beat reporter, but I was kind of lazy about leaving the house at the time. So in theory, maybe I would be the boss of all the beat reporters—breaking stories and bossing everyone around.

Regardless, the Dream was there. I was a *woman* with *something to say*, and I was writing, and I was smoking cigarettes in a way that was fashionable and cool then—that was true about me. But somewhere in the middle of that not-quite-Kerouac-ian, nicotine-clouded, clear-as-day, beautiful and exciting and promising picture of my Life, I got lost.

Several (adult) people brought to my attention that I would be poor as dirt as a writer. It terrified me (more on this later). Looking back, I can't imagine why those statements mattered to me. But it was a bad song with a good beat, an earworm—the sentiment crawled into my head and festered there. *You gonna be poor. You gonna starve. You gonna die.*

Of course, I know why it mattered to me. *Childhood matters.*

And because it matters, I can easily pinpoint one childhood emotion I felt the most: *Fear.*

Fear was an emotion I knew early. Too much, too soon, too fast. Fear around financial security was one of my earliest Fear sets, enhanced later by the Fear of Disappointing Others and the Fear of my body.

My dad was self-employed. Naturally, there was Fear—the Fear of financial devastation, failure, employees, and taxes. I remember the slow-burning undertone about where the next dollar would come from. The sound of the calculator would take on a worrisome, deliberate tenor during these times. The voices raised with other contractors. But I was also entrusted with the information, the burden of it all—directly and unapologetically—like another adult living in the house.

Now the money always came, it seemed. But I did not know how to help. I did not understand that financial talk was just part of adulting and that I (and my nipples) was okay, so I remained trapped in this Fear.

We might not have enough. Never enough. I am not enough. I am disappointing everyone. I am a disappointment.

So when the time came to step into who and what I was supposed to be (the journalist), outsiders tapped into my Fear system: *You won't make any money as a writer. Everyone will be disappointed.* The mere mention of not making money and not having enough for the rest of my Life zapped me.

I was terrified. I promptly put away my little notebook. I knew I couldn't risk it. I needed to choose smarter, to choose a profession where money would never be an issue. Within a week, I had changed my major from journalism to English, the universal degree for "writing is easy for me"—law schools love English majors. Language to study? Well, *Latin* of course.

Fast-forward: I sat in civil procedure class on the first day of law school. I knew with every fiber of my being that this time I had truly chosen wrong. But I also understood and absorbed the absolute pride my family expressed in me sitting there that morning, on the first day of law school. *Must make them proud.*

So, despite the constant low-rumble pooppants pit of my stomach, I stayed in law school.

I fought hard to stay afloat. I did the law school things like trying out for moot court (failed), mock trial (nope), and writing for a legal journal (scored). I graduated, and not at the bottom, either. Somewhere safely hidden in the middle. I developed some confidence that I would not be homeless and unemployed. I would have a roof over my head and a roster of criminal clients to keep me cozy, (also) petrified, and paid. All were proud. All but me.

This is when I really cultivated that serious drinking problem.

Turns out that the actuality of making so serious a Life decision incorrectly was far worse than the prospect of being a dirt-poor writer. The cold-Fear dread of the opposite poles of my dreamed versus chosen Life was emotionally sickening. Only I had no idea at the time that was going on—I buried the lost dream of being a writer as if it never happened. "Moving on! Never happened! Keep going!" I mean, I should be "happy"! Everyone was so proud of me. Proud of me for heading into the esteemed profession of law. Proud of me for doing something difficult. (But also I suspected simultaneously disappointed in me because I was quite overweight and smelled like wine most of the time.) Knowing that I was not meant for law was debilitating. I had picked a career (and a hard one) that could arguably last forty or fifty years, and right out of the gate, I knew it was a mistake.

I would have Enough.

But I had chosen Wrong.

I Knew it.

And in my mind, I had No Choice but to live with it. *You made your bed.*

Lie in it. *All I want to do is lie in bed.*

I was Afraid, and I didn't know how to deal. *I need to escape this feeling.*

So I became a self-burying, body-destroying, emotional-hoarding, binge-eating, self-loathing drunk.

I messed up. I keep messing up. I AM a big effing mistake.

IDENTIFYING THE CORE BELIEFS

Believe it or not, identifying our Core Beliefs is pretty easy. Start by making a list of what you *believe* your Core Beliefs are.

The problem is? Your list is probably garbage.

If you want to dig deep and identify the Core Beliefs that might be driving a crazy train you're riding, then you gotta be a ninja. Because your neat little list might be full of lies.

The second-most effective way to find your beliefs is to listen to the words you say—to yourself.

Some of us may have more voices than others. I have a mean girl named Gladys, and she has the voice of a man. The negative ones are louder, actually easy to spot. If you listen to the mean shit you say to yourself when you're at the low points, the sad points, the hopeless moments—those are some Core Beliefs. Listen to the voices when you are doing a presentation, walking into the gym, leading a meeting, or eating something not so great.

Dismantling some Core Beliefs might feel like a decline into darkness. A bit of chaos, if you will. Chaos which is "the experience of reeling unbound and unsupported through space when your guiding routines and traditions collapse." Sounds like fun, doesn't it?[29]

In my core, I believe that I am huge and slow (and why not, inverted). In the grand scheme of things, who cares if I am huge and slow? No one. No one cares. As a result, I pretend that I also don't care, so I stay fat and slow—in my mind—at whatever weight or speed I am. In other words, I have this belief, and I continue to perpetuate the story in my head—irrespective of what I actually look like or the speed I actually move. I can go out and set a personal record 5K pace, and I still say, "Slow." This way of thinking is a self-destructive pandemic. Because I will never ever be Enough, talking like this. I make it so by believing it so.

What else do I see? Because I carry around the Core Belief that I am hard to love, then I am consequently also unloved and unlovable—and therefore, what am I truly doing here (on this Earth) anyway? *Worthless. Hard to love. Probably because I am huge and slow and inverted. Might as well drive myself into a tree.* As you can see, they all compound into a pile of destructive Core Belief mess.

Some of my positive Core Beliefs?

Even though I had a childhood Fear of scarcity, I have managed to forge a mentality of *Abundance*. This didn't come until recently, but I have managed to cultivate it—and well. I truly believe (e.g., changed a Core Belief to believe) that in my Life I have and will have Enough. I believe I will make Enough money, that I have (and will have) Enough Resources, work hard Enough, and can make the Life I want. I believe I will do this as long as it takes.

Is it because I am "privileged"? I'm sure there's an argument there—someone is bound to make it for me. But my rebuttal would be: Privileged people can still live in a world of scarcity—maybe not in clothes or cars, but in their attitudes, beliefs, and comfort. Scarcity and abundance have nothing to do with financial state; it's a state of mind, an attitude, a way to live, a belief system.

(But having Enough and *being* Enough are different—and I struggle with the latter.)

I managed to overcome a vicious alcohol addiction mostly by deciding to quit. Quitting booze so "easily" begs the question: Why do I still struggle with cookies? Because my Core Beliefs around food and my body are different from those around alcohol. For me, it's that clear (now). It's what I had long believed: I am not meant to be a drunk, but perhaps I am meant to always be a big, unhealthy, slow girl.

While we're at it, here's my favorite piece of useless advice: *Just love yourself as you are! Accept yourself as you are!*

Um, does anyone actually think that people don't want to love themselves? Of course we want to love ourselves, to be loved, to have love everywhere. We have a deep desire to love and accept, but self-love cannot be the starting point for everyone. Many of us feel paralyzed when it comes to loving ourselves because we have a history of believing that we are hard to love. Or we think we are hard to love because we are not smart enough, our parents were abusive, or someone cheated on us. (More on self-love and self-care in Chapter 10.)

Everyone is *something*—some identifiable element of a Core Belief.

We are easily incapacitated by pesky, negative Core Beliefs hidden deep, deep in our souls. We are stuck because we do not speak of them. We push them farther and farther down. Or, we see them, but hate ourselves for thinking them. So we put our heads in the ground, fill our mouths with the sand, and swallow our words. We loathe ourselves for feeling this way, yet we have no idea how to dig out, to stop drowning and start breathing.

We must begin with not only figuring out these Core Beliefs but also being honest about our feelings—our inner, dark, and ugly feelings about ourselves, the world, the people around us, and our past.

We need to bring our Core Beliefs into the light. (Maybe not for the entire world to see but for our own eyes.) We must see them. Without seeing, we cannot begin to love or accept or heal. Without healing, we cannot begin to change. And without change, we cannot experience the Life we are meant to Live.

In order to change, we must break through denial and acknowledge that the issue or problem exists or that the past happened to us: "people don't change what they can't see. And in order to break through their denial, they often have to get a clear picture of what was wrong in their families and the techniques they developed for coping with it."[30] *Addiction. Disordered eating. Personality disorders. Anxiety. Depression. Sexual dysfunction.*

I'm taking a risk in sharing what's next. I know that. But I'm doing it because I want to expose this Core Belief process. And it's a gnarly one.

Deep down in my soul, I think there is nothing worse than ME being fat. There, I said it. Again, I don't care if anyone else is fat. But for me? It's the ultimate symbol of rejection from my past—rejection by my family, my friends, my boyfriends, society, myself.

Am I trying to be a fat shamer? No, hell no. That's my farthest wish.

Is it superficial? You bet your ass it is.

Well, *so now what?* This is precisely the issue.

The paradox: I don't want to be fat, but my actions say otherwise. I mean, I have actively tried to make myself bigger in the past. To be safer, more secure. So no one could kidnap, rape, or assault me. So I would be less afraid. To be bigger so I am stronger. Yet this smallness—this skinniness, this shrinking—is the thing I also want? For the love . . . no wonder I am confused and have been suicidal.

But from someone who has struggled and knows this struggle in *so many women* (and men), I must talk about it. Try and make sense of it. Why is this a hang-up? Why?

Surprise, it comes down to a Core Belief.

Am I okay—if I am fat? Well, I hold a deep belief that the answer is no, because from a young age I was told that was so. I was told that I was fat by kids at school. This alleged Truth was further evidenced by a scale at the doctor's office and lean school box lunches of carrots and cottage cheese packed for me. "Fat" was hinted at by my family, never in a mean way—but more in the recognition that "this child just ate five pieces of pizza at age eight and would have pounded a sixth if we hadn't stopped her." The idea that I was flawed and fat as F was solidified when I was put on a diet alongside my grandmother.

Fat became negative because of what I was told by my family, what society told me, and therefore what I came to believe: fat equals bad.

But even worse—I began to understand (later in Life) that I made myself bigger for a reason. That is why I can share that "fat is bad" for me. Because I made myself this way and for a damn good reason: to draw attention away from my body, to keep parental comments at bay, to keep the world away—I gained weight as a defense mechanism, as a way of hiding from or fighting the world. To protect myself from kidnapping and assault. I still do it. When I am hurt, I go for the fridge. *You don't love me, I'll eat myself sick and make myself not love me too.* When I am angry, I go straight for the pantry. *Time to fight, asshole! I'm fueling up.*

That is why "fat" is toxic for me. Because for me, "fat" is a direct result of not dealing with my shit. Being overweight isn't even about the food or society or my jeans. It's about me bringing my shame, emotions, rage, and Fear into the light—to look at my Truth and deal with it. To figure out where to place the feelings of powerlessness, unworthiness. The Core Belief, while seemingly shallow on the surface, is actually pretty deep and dark.

That being said, we, as a culture, have much work to do in the world of body acceptance. I understand that some people may be upset by my words. *Hell, I am upset by them.* I am angry that at forty years old I am even thinking about body image, for the love! The last thing I want to do is perpetuate this whole societal image issue.

I just want to point out that while we are raging against the media, we might be closer to addressing our own Truth. So I feel with all of my being that I need to rage against it.

Standing in my Truth has been a necessary part of my healing. Without understanding what the Core Beliefs *are*—good or bad—we can't begin to grow and change. By telling my Truth here, I am exposing the process, the way through, out, and beyond. Recognizing the Core Beliefs simply for what they are—without judgment and hatred—is the first step.

This is me telling one of mine.

And maybe someone won't like it. Maybe I'll get Tweeted—that's okay too. I am not writing this blindly; I know what repercussions Truth can have. I have also learned that worrying about what the Other People think is Nonsense.

If we don't like something—we can leave it, change it, or we can accept it.[31] And if we cannot accept it—and that is okay too—time to change it. See how that works?

I am not telling anyone to change themselves or their bodies; that is not the point at all. If you are at a place of acceptance and that You are Enough, that's amazing and powerful.

But if you want to change yourself, your body, or your beliefs, that is okay too. You are allowed.

Walking around blinded by our Core Beliefs is part of the Nonsense that keeps building more Nonsense. At some point, we must admit what's going on back there and how we freaking feel. We must admit that we have been exposed to less-than-ideal situations—and as a result, we have yucky, gross, and embarrassing Core Beliefs.

I wanted to continue to use this Core Belief ("fat is the worst, I am fat and always will be, and therefore, I am also the worst") as a convenient excuse to not show up for Life, to say I was a failure, as a foolproof plan to "prove" why I was hard to love, slow, worthless.

My Core Belief was serving the purpose I needed it to—in order to prove that I was hard to love. But I don't need that particular Core Belief anymore. So I continue to work to change these things—on my terms.

KNOW THYSELF

When I was in the last throes of giving birth to my son, the midwife brought in a huge floor-length mirror and asked, "Do you want to watch your son being born?"

I swear I might have screamed, "Fuck no!" in the middle of the delivery room.

I know myself just fine, thanks.

Emotional Intelligence and doing what the Delphic Oracle says ("Know Thyself"), however, is like giving birth in front of a mirror. We are turning the insides out and seeing everything for what it is.

Knowing Thyself need not be some form of humiliation, but it is a form of authenticity and reality. Lauren Handel Zander, author of the book *Maybe It's You*, recommends not only standing in your Truth but telling all of your Truths and eradicating the lies—by telling those lies also. *Admitting your lies.* I will admit I break out in a special hive when I think about exposing all my skeletons to the world. I refuse to do it. I have spoken to Lauren on several occasions, and I tell her, "You can take your lie list and shove it up your ass." She laughs and says, "But then you will be free." *Ah.*

When I was in college, I received an email giving me "Free $100" to play blackjack online. Online gambling was fairly new and shiny, and I had no freaking idea that it was addicting. With a pint of vodka and a Bjork disc on repeat, I managed to blow $900 in one evening. I worked at a smoothie shop and knew that I would need to steal smoothies or learn to launder money if I kept that up.

So I quit gambling, but I continued drinking.

I find it strange that I knew myself enough to know that a Life of gambling and stealing was not particularly something I wanted. However, drinking alcohol did not seem as obvious. Why was that a permissible form of sabotage for me? Why didn't I know myself enough to walk away from drinking—something that was clearly becoming an issue?

I wasn't living my Purpose. So what was I doing? Not living my Life either. Gary John Bishop said that finding a Purpose is bullshit— that we only have the here and now. Wherever you are, *that* is your Purpose and you should be in your Life. Live! I tend to agree with myself . . . and GJB.* Regardless: I was not living any Purpose at the time. I was not Living at all.[32]

And I knew it. So once I started drinking, I kept going. I did not feel any stigma about it.

Little by little, my drinking grew crazy. I could easily pour a giant cup of orange juice and vodka and be obliterated out of my mind. I would download songs on Napster all night long. (On dial-up, y'all. I had over five thousand songs on dial-up. Figure that out.) I read my books for class sober, and then I poured the first drink when I needed to write papers—and I would turn them in, not knowing a crack about what I wrote.

I got to the point where I didn't write a paper unless inebriated. As such, I wrote ballsy, outlandish papers. I got A's. I would turn the paper in, forget about it, then receive it back from the professor (when I was sober) and think, "Who wrote this?" I never remembered writing them, but damn, some of them were really, really good. I had a certain virtuosity in drunk writing. I was brave; I was free. And therefore, I used booze as a necessity for writing.

Learning to Know Thyself myself was hard. I missed the memo somewhere in Life about learning who I was, what I wanted, and developing the tools to get there.

I didn't think that I could do Life sober. Perhaps it was because I produced my best, most praised writing when I was off-the-wall drunk. Maybe that Success was part of the addiction. I know there was something powerful about writing completely unencumbered. Truth can be in booze; but that's about where the benefits end. *Emotional Intelligence gets better with age.*

---

* After my podcast conversation with Gary John Bishop, I changed my perspective a bit on the idea of "Purpose." (Should tell you how convincing that guy is.) Instead of always seeking out our magical "Purpose," we need to focus more on LIVING our lives. Our current Life is our Purpose. *Now is the time to Live.* (See introduction.)

During that time period and for almost twenty years after, I did not believe that I could pull off any stroke of genius on my own without booze. I had a fundamental belief that I could not do it. But as I got older—I thought, *Wait a second.* That was some Emotional Intelligence pulling its head out of the sand. I was challenged with many things after getting sober, but writing was a big one. Learning to write (anything) sober was like learning to walk again.

Self-awareness, if it's not a skill we naturally possess, is definitely a skill that can get easier the older we get. (Although I have plenty of experience with older individuals who have absolutely no self-awareness. You can see them fighting Life, fighting themselves, fighting every system and in a constant state of "being wronged." Remember that a lack of self-awareness may "bring on inner turmoil." Self-awareness has absolutely nothing to do with anyone else.)

Self-awareness is recognizing that we are developing a gambling problem and are seriously hindered by booze—and that these things are not "okay." Not even from a financial or legal sense but from a sense of self—that's what matters. Self-awareness is an ability that forces us to feel all the feels, all the emotions, all day—to take a step back and say, "I'm making a stinking mess of things" or "I need to stop __."

When we are aware of ourselves and we can see, then we can feel.

BUT WE DON'T WANT TO FEEL

No one wants to feel all the feels, the hurts and pains, the rejection, and yet the feels are must-haves. Feels exist. We don't want to feel the feels, so we learn to numb. Instead of harnessing the power of (or cultivating) self-awareness, we retreat to the sand, stick our head in, and pretend like everything is okay—or if it isn't, that the feels aren't happening (let's numb!)—or, that we are just batshit crazy. *I can't deal with this. Now or ever. I will make myself blissfully unaware somehow by taking on some Nonsense behaviors to cope.* Except, bad news: turns out there's no bliss.

We're trying to soothe ourselves like giant babies, because we can't deal. As adults, we can't really suck our thumbs or hold our blankies, so we learn to numb with the available mechanisms: booze and food and affairs and drugs and social media and shopping and porn and whatever else we can do to extreme and silly, self-destructive excess behind closed doors to somehow help hide the wound, unfeel the feelings, dig deep into the sand. And yes, we're all doing it—to some degree.

What if at the same time on the first Monday in June every year, we all stood up and shouted our addictions, eccentricities, and freak-iness—all of the lies in our lives—out loud, for everyone to hear. What if it was no big deal, and we understood that everyone would admit their crazy truths and failures and faults, and then we would all nod and say, "Yep, also me" (or "Not me, but totally get it"), and then we would work to understand that we are all doing the best we can? What if we all just admitted that we have these things in our lives that are messy and destructive but at the same time serve an incredible Purpose? That we aren't weak or flawed or ugly because we struggle? That we are simply trying to unfeel the feelings or meet other needs that are tied to perhaps sadness, regret, loneliness, Fear.

Dealing with my alcohol problem, I somehow intuited that I wasn't pathetic or weak because drinking had such a hold on me. Rather, I *drank for a reason*. The reason? Well, Life is hard, soul-sucking work can be debilitating, parenthood is ridiculous, people can be assholes, and alcohol can serve a very specific purpose: *escape* and *sleepiness*. Also, my childhood (yes, sorry—but there it is again. *Childhood matters*.)

When I drank, I could give two shits about anything—past, present, or future—that was the point, I guess. *Escape*. But there was a tipping point for me—as there is for any excess—because we are not using the substance or the action in a reasonable way. We are using it as a cure-all, a panacea for fixing our supposed cracks, our alleged brokenness. We are using it to numb and cope with abuse, shame, and Fear. When we realize that the behavior just causes more problems (illness, money spent, fights with family, hangovers, weight gain, loss of productivity), we are too far in. We now rely on our habit, behavior, or addiction to get us through each day.

We need it. It's our blankie.

Self-awareness won't cure these numbing tendencies and mechanisms—because remember, we are doing these things for a reason and we don't want to feel. Self-awareness and reframing our Core Beliefs will not stop the desire to numb. It won't cure the so-called benefits we receive from not dealing with our problems.

But once we are aware of certain parts of the past, Beliefs, Truths, lies, tendencies, and numbing—we know them. Our head is out of the sand—even if just a little—like the eyes, a nostril, and one ear. We may not know or understand everything that happened, but we know something did—and that is enough to begin to heal, to change.

This place is where recovery is born. Recovery from the past, pain, addiction, or destructive behavior starts with the reality of the present—where we are, *and* where we were. It begins with asking yourself the right questions and answering them truthfully. Mental Health is a commitment to reality.[33]

As such, because Truth and reality are hard and full of pain, we like to avoid them. "We can revise our maps only when we have the discipline to overcome that pain. . . . Conversely, we must always consider our personal discomfort relatively unimportant and, indeed, even welcome it in the service of the search for truth. Mental Health is an ongoing process of dedication to reality at all costs."[34]

Once we know the *reasons* why we are doing the destructive things we do—all the binge eating, obsessive exercising, ridiculous amounts of porn, drinking, or (and?) cheating on a spouse—then we can begin to figure out a way to stop doing them. The destructive things are merely coping mechanisms. Nonsense is a coping mechanism—that's all. And once we recognize that simple fact, we begin to find a way to the other side: to freedom, to healing.

WHY NAMES HURT

A few years ago, it was fun to call myself a "Hot Mess." After all, I had sort of taken on that persona. I believed myself to be klutzy, messy, sloppy, and silly—like Bridget Jones.

But the truth of the matter is that I actually pulled off amazing things in spite of myself, irrespective of my past, my size, my klutzy nature. Cool, right? Sure. Except that I had gone along with a name— Hot Mess.

"Mess" is defined as "a person or thing in a dirty, untidy, or disordered condition." I am certain that I am not dirty—as a person. I am also not untidy—as a person. I am also not in a *disordered condition*. Now, can I be? Sure, sometimes. Is my house? Well, no comment on that.

But just like I *have* fat, I also *have* mess. I *am* not mess.

Likewise, you are not a Hot Mess. Despite what you feel or think or believe, you are not a mess. You might *have* some mess. You might have some *fat*. You might be a little drunk or feel lonely. But you are not Mess, and you are not Fat. You are not a Drunk, and you are not Alone.

From a starting point, I want you to rewind to the Core Beliefs and think of some of the labels you have given yourself.

When I was little, my dad called me "Bear." It came from the simple fact that my skin would turn dark brown during the summer, and (I suspect that) I looked like a little (chubby) bear cub. As I grew, I actually liked being "Bear." My weightlifting[*] teammates picked it up from a meet where my dad screamed, "Let's go, Bear!" *Bear*. Well, it

---

[*] I competed in the sport of Olympic weightlifting from ages thirteen to nineteen. My mom desperately wanted a ballerina for a daughter. She got a weightlifter. So I sometimes wear a tutu when I lift to make her smile.

was an animal and a persona I could get behind. Bears are strong, big animals. They love fish and will fight when necessary. They take care of their cubs. Additionally, bears are very gentle and extremely tolerant of other animals. Bears also roll over huge rocks and logs in search of food. In fact, they have been known to bend open car doors and pry open windshields to get to food.[35] I have totally felt that way before.

The value of a Name is incredibly important. Whether you call yourself Bear or Hot Mess matters. Names, like childhood and likely a part of childhood, matter.

As we grow up, we learn intuitively about the power of words. We learn from little jerks named Chris who call us *fatty-fatty two-by-four*. Or the absolute worst: *Is that a bra?* screamed from across the playground in fourth grade. Yes! To hide my inverted nipples, you little shit.

Words are powerful. Forever-burned words leave scars and create echoes and trajectories for years. The Butterfly Effect.

I don't love you anymore.

You will never be _____.

I am so sorry for your loss.

You are not my friend.

You have disappointed me.

You will always be alone.

I am leaving you.

It's cancer.

You are getting fat.

I will never forgive you.

Who do you think you are?

There is power in Names and naming, and as Dr. Rachael Peckham, associate professor of English at Marshall University, acknowledges, "Where there is power, there is potential for problems."[36]

Peckham explained to me, "Naming can be both productive and destructive. With regard to naming, it's incredibly complicated. Naming always exists in a context and it bears great power. The beautiful thing, however, is that through changing our names, our nicknames, our self-descriptions, we have the power to redefine ourselves. Language can be a prison if we allow it. At the same time, we can use words and names to break out and be free."

Words are important. Maybe we can't control what Other People call us. Sometimes employing cruel Names or nicknames is a weak-minded exertion of their power. But we can control the words that we use for ourselves.

Many of us know the value of words—but only intuitively. Taking a moment to absorb the power of words is in part learning to identify Nonsense. On a planet where words hold such power, bullying and hate speech are ways to assert a messed-up version of authority over others. When children are cruel on the playground, they are simply but effectively singling out the "weak" to make themselves more powerful. When the bullies emerge in middle school to mock the clothing and hair of their classmates? Same deal. Mean kids and bullies aren't limited to adolescence. Our culture has somehow accepted that kids will be kids—but when those kids grow up to be word slingers on social media and abusive in work environments, we realize we are living in one giant playground.

We feel the power of words spoken by others. We know the power we have by the things we say to others. In Chapters 6 and 7, we will learn how to navigate the waters of Other People, relationships, and the like. But the recognition and quest for a Year of No Nonsense starts with us. The words we speak to ourselves first. The Names we call ourselves and allow ourselves to be called. The internal monologue that we play on repeat. That is first.

For now, I want you to make a note of the Names that you give yourself, the Names you have been given by others.

I had a phone call with my first real boyfriend the other day. He owns a landscaping company in my hometown, and I was coordinating some yard cleanup for my mother-in-law. He and I had a nice chat, but before we hung up, he said, "Thanks, Mere!" With those two words, I was catapulted to another place and time. He was the first one to call me "Mere." The way he used to say it— well, there was a playful cadence to it—and I heard it again. He was a fun boyfriend. I liked him. And all that with a quick "Thanks, Mere."

All with a word, a Name.

If something as small as that can generate a kind of response, what kind of cosmic reaction do I have to "bitch" or "fatty-fatty"? The negative words? The hurtful Names? We might not want to admit how big an impact they make. The problem, too, is that sometimes we hear the Names so often that we no longer have a reaction. We have accepted them as Truth. We have blessed them as our Names. That is the great undoing that must happen. We must unravel the Names we do not want. They are not ours to carry.

You are not a Hot Mess. You are not any of the things on your list of Names that you do not want to be. Keep the good ones. Keep the ones that give you energy and power. If you're a Bear (and wanna be one), then be a bear. Let's get rid of the rest. How? Well, I'll be honest, it's fairly simple.

Change the Name. Write it down. Pick a warrior name, in the style of the movie *Fried Green Tomatoes*. Just don't ram your car repeatedly into another car in the parking lot. Reinvent yourself. This is the time.

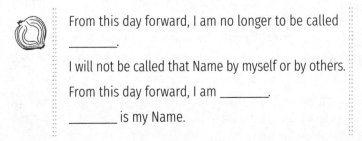

From this day forward, I am no longer to be called
_____.
I will not be called that Name by myself or by others.
From this day forward, I am _____.
_____ is my Name.

Maybe this "new" Name is simply your real Name.

Maybe you change your real Name. Did you know that if you hate your birth name, you can change it? Relatively easily in most states with the help of a lawyer and even online legal forms?

Summary: If we don't like something, we can sometimes easily change it.

You can't control what people say behind your back, so quit even thinking about it. But you can tell people what to call you to your face. For the most part, when we tell someone to stop calling us something— they often do. If they love us, they will stop. If these folks insist on calling you something you hate, then it may be time for some bigger actions, some new friends, new scenery, different relationships.

We inadvertently give the Other People the power of naming us. It's time to change the Names you dislike. Time to change the Names you call yourself. Names can hurt. Pick ones that don't.

WHY NUMBERS HURT

I just had the fun experience of my yearly trip to the gynecologist.

I saw a little chart on the counter. The dreaded BMI chart. BMI stands for "body mass index," and it takes your height and weight (only) and decides whether you are underweight, healthy weight, overweight, obese, or "morbidly obese."

I took a picture and posted on social media, joking, "Still obese!" with an eye roll.[*] My post almost immediately received the expected reaction: "This chart sucks!" and "I won't be defined by this ancient chart!" *Good, that's how I feel too.*

So, I had my lovely pelvic exam (who doesn't love stirrups?), and the doctor (whom I adore) left the room for me to get dressed.

---

[*] The BMI chart should be used only to assess completely inactive people who have zero muscle mass (if it should be used at all).

When she came back in, she looked at me apologetically and said, "This is a big corporate hospital, and I hate that. But I have to give you this."

"What is it?" I asked.

She handed me a piece of paper. "It's your BMI information," she said. "I know you work out and eat well. So disregard it. But I have to check the box."

I laughed and smiled, brushing it off. *Obese.*

But as she walked out of the room, I could feel my face get hot and a wave of shame rush over me. I was gutted. And I can admit that is a dumb thing to get gutted over, especially since I know that I am doing everything within my power to eat well and take care of myself and that BMI actually stands for "bullshit measurement index." My recent bloodwork was fantastic, and I am healthy as a horse. I should have laughed, brushed it off, and meant it.

But it hurt.

Why? Because on some planet we all decided that Numbers matter—big time. That we are defined, likeable, or more valuable based on our weight, cholesterol, IQ, SAT scores, paycheck, social media followers, number of pets or children or spouses, cars and homes, rental properties, and vacations taken. We are all counting, watching, and looking at ourselves; then we look up the Numbers of the Other People around us, and we compare.

Some Numbers matter, just like some words matter. For instance, a heartbeat of zero is super-important information, along with "Next Stop, Station 10" when you needed Station 4. But like naming and words, we need to put Numbers into their proper places.

 We are not defined by the Names we have been given; we are not defined by the Numbers in our lives.

My late grandmother, Mombow, and I joined Weight Watchers in 1990. I was turning eleven years old the summer before sixth grade and gaining weight like gangbusters. I was also starting puberty. Somehow that was not taken into consideration.

I remember being at a WW meeting with Mombow. I had lost eleven pounds to date, but we both had gained that week. I remember that shame spelled out in my little weigh-in diary like it was yesterday. Green ink with smeared, sloppy handwriting revealed that I had gained three pounds. I remember thinking, "Now, I have only lost eight." Mombow had gained a similar amount.

I was 111 pounds. She was 211. One hundred pounds separated us.

We gained the weight, so we went out for pizza after the meeting ("just this once" and we would "start tomorrow"). I liked her. Correction: I *loved* her. *She and I are the same*, I thought.

She said something at dinner that I will never forget. "Meredith, some people have willpower and some people don't. That's why we are going to Weight Watchers, because we don't have any."

I nodded with understanding, even though I was confused. *How was I not born with willpower?* That seemed really unfair.

I knew I needed help with my body, but only because people told me I did. *My body was weird. Inverted. My body was fat.* I had known that for some time. I was ashamed of everything from my "such a pretty face" down to the *inverted* situation, and I had been for years. Weight Watchers was something that could help me—this willpowerless child with such a pretty face.

I was glad I had Mombow—she was the only one "like" me that I knew.

I was made to believe that I could learn willpower. So I believed that. But willpower might have been the lie all along. Willpower is a crossroads of what we want and how much we are willing to sacrifice to get it. I was confused about what I (personally) wanted—because I was a child (!) who liked food, and I didn't know that I was oh-so flawed. I did, however, realize the lengths that my family would have to travel in order to have a nonportly kid.

I didn't have a strong enough reason to not eat. I liked food. I was a child, for the love. I didn't care enough, because deep down I loved food more than I cared about what my body looked like—especially at a young age. It didn't matter to me, because again, I was a kid. So with the dieting, I was just trying to be what they said I should—to make my family happy, to look like my very thin, long-legged mother, despite my squishy belly and short legs. *People pleaser.*

Mombow and I quit Weight Watchers soon after.

Weight Watchers couldn't help me. Therefore, I was unhelp-able, I thought. I didn't have willpower. I wasn't born with it. WW didn't give it to me. I would always be "fat," and "nothing worked," and "oh well."

Looking back on Mombow, who passed away in 2016, I think about willpower and I smile. Turns out that she had some of the biggest feats of will and power in the world. She was relentless with her money and saved every single penny beyond what she needed. She worked at her job with pride—in a time when many women didn't work at all.

But with food? Eh. This "willpower" that she believed she lacked went out the window.

Toward the end, she didn't eat much at all, and was the tiniest version of Mombow I had ever imagined. As she got sick, her mind and body changed, and food was not a thing for her. Eating was something that no one could get her to do, as is often the case in declining Health.

Suddenly that mysterious battle with food was so insignificant and had nothing to do with will or power—the end was about *Life* and *love*. When she died she was probably 111 pounds. I was 211.

As with our Names, we might need to reformulate the importance of our Numbers. Some numbers are *Nonsense* (to us). Other Numbers are great indicators of our own Nonsense. But as a starting point, we might want to take Numbers like body weight and social media followers and put them in the box where they belong—a box of data points that can be charted, not a box of soul points that describe who we *are*. BMI: bullshit measurement index.

Does this mean that we should ignore all Numbers? No. Physics and math* are real, and body weight does matter—if you want to qualify for the Boston Marathon or do strict pull-ups. But even still it's not an absolute: I look at body weight as a *probability indicator*. Body weight tells us our odds of being able to do certain things. The Number on the scale does not prove whether or not we can or can't accomplish something. I know plenty of lightweight folks who can't do a pull-up or run a marathon. It often comes down to willingness to work and perhaps the unwillingness to let other things define us.

As Reuben Meerman points out in his famous TedX talk, "The Mathematics of Weight Loss," the only difference between washboard abs and a six-pack stomach is $C_{55}H_{104}O_6$—or the chemical compound of a fat molecule.[37] Some have more of these and some less.

Your body weight should not stop you from putting your Life into orbit. Instead of thinking about that scale, let's contemplate how badass the Universe is to actually hold us on a planet, how wondrous our bodies are to breathe and move and function.[38]

Who cares what the Numbers are? We are magnificent! (Do a little dance about that!)

Put all Numbers in their places, as data points—nothing more, nothing less.

---

* But even in astrophysics, the measurement of gravity (called "Big G") is known as a "finicky" number. Whereas Big G as a number is hugely important for cosmology and modeling the universe, the number admittedly doesn't have any *practical* benefits here on Earth. The fact that scientists and physicists do not know "Big G with perfect precision didn't stop us from putting a man on the Moon, or from plotting the paths of satellites." I mean, if those guys don't care about Big G's precision . . . why in the hell do we?

People defy the odds all the time—be one of those people, no matter what the Names or Numbers say.

· · · · **Checkpoint 2** ·

1. What are two Core Beliefs you hold? How have these Beliefs shaped you for the good or not-so-good?

2. What causes you shame right now? Make a short list. How does this list tie in to your Core Beliefs? Are they related at all?

3. Thinking about Names that you have been called—are there any you want to adopt? Do away with? Keep a positive one, or pick a "warrior" name, and fill in the blanks:
   From *this day forward, I am no longer to be called* _____, *by myself or by others.*
   I am _____.
   _____ *is my Name.*

4. Extra credit: List all your Core Beliefs that you can think of. Put a check by those that have impacted you for the good. Put an X next to those that have caused you harm or could really use a change or update.

#PositiveCoreBeliefs #BeABear #YearOfNoNonsense

3

Breaking Up with the Lies We Have Been Told

SINCE THE BEGINNING OF OUR LIVES, WE'VE BEEN LIED TO. LIES MAY not always come from bad places, but lies are happening, and they are flying fast and furiously. They are told by our parents, our teachers, our friends, the government, the media, our employers and coworkers, and people on Instagram. If our pets could lie, they would too. By the way, we also lie to ourselves. A lot. By lying to ourselves, we are also lying to everyone else around us.

The depth of all the lies and omissions allows us to understand that some of our current state is not totally our fault. At the same time, we can see what is our fault. Which begs the question of whether we truly need to beat ourselves up for one more thing. Probably not. But we do have responsibility in it all—and that sucks.

After all, we came into this world blameless and perfect—just as we were. We were little blobs of baby at some point, and then we had flawed humans raise us in a flawed world, sending us off to flawed teachers and schools in a flawed country with flawed leaders and media, working for flawed bosses and paying taxes to the flawed man.

If we look at our lives on that plane, how did we even have a chance to get anything right? It's not our fault, right?

Sounds good and logical to me.

So let's start with blame.

BLAME

Under the method of "blame effectively," we can expel a few things from our lives, our histories. We are empowered to lay out the Truth of the messed-up parts of our Lives via perhaps good old-fashioned blame. But we are also required to recognize (and be grateful for) how even those horrific, messed-up things, experiences, and people helped shape us—for the good. And if not for the good, for at least the place we are.

This is the paradox I mentioned in the beginning, about childhood—that sometimes Life is not black-and-white. Even the bad can have some good to it, and both the good and the bad can exist about the same situation and experience. Yes, for many of us that may be a tough pill to swallow. It might feel too soon. We may mentally shut down. I get it, I do. Abuse (the wide gamut), neglect, violence, sickness, pain, and other unmentionable wrongs done to us[*] or against us may seem impossible to be grateful for. It might feel like a long shot to be grateful for our addictions, our "weaknesses," and our regrets.

I look at my Life. As much as I had some not-so-great childhood stuff, hated being a lawyer, struggled with alcohol, and still struggle with body image, I am grateful for it all—because without a story to tell, I wouldn't have . . . well, a story to tell.

---

[*] By people who were supposed to love us, to boot. That's the hard thing to overcome.

I loved an article I read on *Medium* in which the author talked about blaming *alcohol* for her *alcohol addiction* as the key to her sobriety.[1] I, too, think I came to sobriety blaming the actual *booze*—and blaming it effectively. *This is YOUR fault, you piece of shit bottle of wine.*

We can learn something with every single hurt and harm if we are willing to blame productively, effectively. Also, it's important to recognize who or what is to blame. *You are a jerk for beating me the way you did, and YOU beating ME was YOUR fault. But I am not going to give YOU another second of power.*

Take the blame and place it where it's due. It's not your fault you were abused—it's your family member's fault. It's not your fault that you developed a two-decade booze habit—it's the fault of the wine (and the family member who beat you—you needed to escape that memory).

That is not your fault, but it will be your fault if you don't figure out the next step, the way to move on.

And to do that, we must take away the power of the harm(er)— whether it's a substance, a person, or an institution. We can allow the blame to wash from us and move the energy toward healing our wounds.

Can we thank a person who harmed us? Or thank a thing that we were (are) addicted to? Can we align our hearts and our minds to something that foreign? Can we reconcile the treatment we received with the holes in our souls?

We can—because that thing (or those things) has made us the strong, resilient people we are. We can move past it all, and we must.

Because no matter what evil or horrible thing has happened, we are here. We are alive. And as long as we are alive, we can do something. We can learn to put blame in its place. We can put the lies and the Truth in their places. And then we can move forward.

Now . . . on to the lies.

LIE #1: YOU WILL *NEVER* BE / YOU *ARE* / YOU WILL *ALWAYS* BE

One of the most insidious lies is the one that tells us what we *are* or will *always* be or will *never* become.

This type of lie originates when we are young: *You will never become a rocket scientist. You are lazy. You will always be bad at math.* In the case of Pluto, *you are no longer a planet.* Whatever the statement, we may have accepted it as Truth delivered by an authority figure (parents, teachers, coaches, church leaders). Then we began to act (or not act) upon the false Truth (believing it to be actually true), and the whole damn thing spiraled from there.

Only the few of us who had superior emotional intelligence for our ages or BS-sleuthing wherewithal to reject these statements have overcome the potential obstacles the statements created. Unfortunately, many of us don't realize that rejecting the insanity is a choice when we are young—because we don't know we are experiencing said insanity or we aren't strong enough to withstand the punishment of rejecting the insanity. Again, we trusted where the messages were coming from. Then we don't rage against the proverbial or actual man until later in Life (if at all).

(Like, if I were Pluto, I would now say, "Bitch, please. I am a planet.")

I had a middle school coach who informed me that I would never be a runner. I admittedly wasn't a fast or skilled runner. But I worked hard in sports, because that's what I knew to do. After a game (in which I was running, working hard), the coach muttered, "Lord, girl, you're never going to be a runner if you run like that."

If I run like WHAT? Like me? I was floored. Wait a fresh damn second here. I was just out there running! What do you mean that I will "never be" a runner? I am running! I was running!

I knew that running *felt* hard, but I did it anyway. I kept going. I moved a little slower than some of my teammates, but I got the job done. I had Hustle. I had drive. I tried, for the love.

But this coach was an authority figure, so I took what was said as Truth. *Well, I will never be a runner. Alrighty, then.*

Later, when the opportunity to become a weightlifter arose, I thought, "Well here's a sport with zero running. Since I will never be a runner, I should probably throw myself wholeheartedly into this thing."

The weightlifting coach said, "Meredith is really strong," and because he said that, I believed it. And I still believe it.

However, if the weightlifting coach had told me, "You're so weak, you make my coffee look strong. Go back to running," then God knows where I would be. Chasing my tail, shit-faced drunk, somewhere between a track and a barbell.

I clung to this *positive* belief: I am strong. Thus, I became stronger. I stepped into exactly who the coaches said I was. *I will never be a runner. But I will always be strong.* We often do just that—good, bad, or ugly.

Stepping into beliefs, therefore, can be powerful or destructive. So when a belief has a negative or destructive power, like "you will never be a runner," true Grit and growth happen when we question or challenge that belief. When I took a look at the statement about running—years and years later when I found triathlon—I decided I would not accept that as an ultimate Truth anymore.

As hard work, Hustle, and Grit would later prove, it turns out that I was a runner too.

OUR SCRIPTS

Other People and experiences may put ideals, ideas, and thoughts into our heads, but we, ultimately, are the ones who drive those principles home. We create and Live our story. We are shaped by the authority figures in our Lives. We deem their words as Truth, and we step into those "Truths" in some way—or in many ways. Don't believe it? Just watch young kids at a political rally. They have no idea what is going on—they are doing exactly what their parents are doing. And later, that eighteen-year-old voter might be voting based off the rally from twelve years ago.

If the Other People interaction was positive, we can accept it, embody it, and run with it. To this day, I believe I am strong. But I have fought tooth and nail to believe *I am a runner* after decades of believing I was not.

We do not intentionally screw ourselves out of confidence, opportunities, and Success from a young age. We do not consciously perpetuate that silliness, but yet, perpetuating it, nonetheless, we are. And by doing so, we totally bend over and take it from ourselves— over and over again. *Why do we say mean things to ourselves? Why is our brain the only real battlefield many of us will encounter?*

We do these things because impressions were made on us when we were too young to know they were shitty impressions. *It's not our fault.* But whoops—now we know (or we are coming to know, little by little)—so now we see, and now we have a responsibility to ourselves to change this situation.

We can change the script.

My friend Susan once said to me, "You are reading the same crappy script over and over again. 'I am overweight. I am slow. I am a miserable lawyer and I will always be that way.' For some reason you keep hanging on to it, replaying it over and over again. Maybe you edit it a little for your blog audience, but at the end of the day—it's the same story. You need to do a full rewrite."

I'll be honest that her assessment of me made me mad. I didn't like being boiled down to a simple thing such as "you are reading your same damn script." I did not like that she hit the nail on the head either. Much like I didn't like it when my husband left me the "get your shit together" note.

"I do not have a script," I huffed to myself. "This is my Life!" Then I turned to page 104 of my not-script-script and continued reading. *Why am I so fat? Why can't I have a job that I love? Why is everything so much harder for me?*

Oh.

For the first time I saw that I did indeed have a script. The script was written out of the culmination of my past experiences—good and bad. I didn't have a thing to do with the original script. It had been crafted from my childhood, from experiences with my parents, bullies, ex-boyfriends, and jerks; from positives and negatives. I didn't write it, but I *was* the one who continued reading it, out loud, to everyone who would listen, over and over again.

We choose whether or not to continue to read that script out loud. We choose whether to change it, from this day forward.

I needed to change my sad-ass script. So I began to tear it up, piece by piece, year by year. I still don't have it rewritten perfectly, but I do know that once I tore up the sad, long, and whiny script—things began to change. I asked myself how I wanted to change. I dared to ask myself what I wanted in Life.

I took "you will never" and "you are not" and "you are" and flipped them into words to be used for good, for progress toward my goals. You too can take the negative script words and add what you *want to believe* and what *you will do*. You can take the BS phrases and make them powerful.

I WILL NEVER . . .

- be a manipulative spouse.
- allow myself to be treated that way again.
- use methamphetamine.

I AM NOT . . .

- a pushover.
- taking one more second of this treatment.
- meant for this job—I can do better.

I AM . . .

- strong.
- a runner.
- a badass Truth teller.

You can decide what you will never be. You can decide who you are. That is your prerogative and your script to write. Just make sure that you choose what is best for you—don't follow the script someone else wrote for you.

LIE #2: HAPPINESS IS THE DESTINATION

How many times have you heard, "You deserve to be happy"?

History has proven to me that choosing anything based on a current "Happiness" state is the wrong decision. This "you deserve to be happy" statement is kinda Nonsense.

I dug myself out of some dark places and dank caves over the last decade. But in reality, I was still hanging out at the cave entrance like a smoker outside a tattoo parlor. I was never too far out into the light. I found it easy to retreat back into the dark-place-tattoo-parlor and continue inking my defunct script onto my wasteland of a body.

I am amazing . . . on paper. On paper. On paper.

Almost six years after I had started this seemingly never-ending search for a better me through exercise and Health and triathlon, I still didn't have my act together. I was not pursuing my passion for work. My desire to do anything related to physical activity was waning. I still was not "happy"—not even close. I continued to beat myself up for the way I looked, the speed I ran, and the piles of regret that were starting to build from what I liked to call "a bit of a drinking problem."

What was going on? What was this path to Happiness? Was Happiness a destination, or was it a frame of mind? If either, then how did I get to either the frame of mind or the destination? Was I just flawed? Was I exceptionally ungrateful? (Totally possible despite gratitude journaling, dips in gratefulness exercises, and the like. I felt like I should be grateful for it all—my current Life, my childhood—but my insides screamed otherwise.) I also dared to ask myself this question: Was I the type of person who just simply wasn't ever going to be Happy?

I considered all of the above as true possibilities.

Money can't buy Happiness. Happiness comes from the inside. Happiness is gratitude. Happiness is ice cream.

But truly, I believe that Happiness is the version of "Happyness" from the movie *The Pursuit of Happyness*:

> It was right then that I started thinking about Thomas Jefferson on the Declaration of Independence and the part about our right to life, liberty, and the pursuit of happiness. And I remember thinking how did he know to put the pursuit part in there? That maybe happiness is something that we can only pursue and Maybe we can actually never have it. No matter what. How did he know that?[2]

Just like Life isn't a destination, Happiness isn't a destination. Happiness was never a destination. We could never, and we still can't, drive there and stay there.

That hard-to-pin-down state we are searching for isn't Happiness at all. We think we are looking for Happiness, but we just want comfort, peace, quiet in our souls, a little internal harmony. (And maybe ten minutes without hearing our names called from somewhere in the house—or the worst: tiny, sticky fingers poking under the bathroom door.)

So peace is perhaps that destination we are seeking. Peace is a more productive, longer-lasting, arguably permanent state. Peace is not emotional; Happiness is pure emotion. Peace is a body-and-mind state of contentment. Happiness is temporary (hooray-type) joy— Happiness is an emotional by-product of peace, contentment, and safety. It comes and goes. And we have been lied to about Happiness our whole lives. *You deserve to be happy. Marriage will make me happy. Children will make me happy. This job will make me happy. Losing weight will make me happy. Winning the world championships in whatever will make me happy.*

All of the above contain kernels of hidden Truth: marriage and children *can* make you happy—some of the time. But marriage and children will make you insane in the worst ways too. A job *can* make you happy—sometimes. But that's a tough one. I have landed many "dream jobs"—and hey, look, I work at none of those places now.

We are not, as humans, wired to be perpetually happy. Quite the opposite, really. "Dissatisfaction with the present and dreams of the future are what keep us motivated. . . . [P]erpetual bliss would completely undermine our will to accomplish anything at all. . . . Recognizing that happiness exists, and that it's a delightful visitor that never overstays its welcome, may help us appreciate it more when it arrives."[3]

Searching for the elusive destination of Happiness is leaving our joy up to external circumstances, people, and things. Happiness is a temporary buzz or an experience, but peace is something we can cultivate, something we have; we can internalize peace, hold on to, and turn to it—when times are hard, we can even lean toward it. Peace is about simply being—and being okay just *being*. Peace is setting ourselves on a path that includes moments and even long streaks of Happiness but doesn't depend on external validation, people, or events to make us whole.

Peace is a state that nurtures our forever-self—the version of ourselves that we strive to become and be—that is the end game. Peace is safety in our bodies and hearts—*that* state *is* the forever goal, the destination. Peace is a sense of calm, contentment, and "okayness" with ourselves and the world, a way to stay grounded, grateful, and calm—no matter how long the journey of Life may be and what challenges—or Happiness—might come (or go) along the way.

Don't let the lie of Happiness drive your Life or your goals.

LIE #3: YOU CAN HAVE IT ALL

I want to be uberclear on my view of "Life is about balance" from the outset. I would hate to mislead you.

So here goes: *Balance is bullshit.*

When I received the "get your shit together" note, I was winning the parenting game on social media, but I was disconnected from my children—for many reasons—mostly the time-crunch of Life. Marriage was okay—that was about it. I cared (sort of) about the food I put in my body but not the alcohol. I had lost a little weight and was keeping it off. Sometimes. But I would regress in body and mind for weeks on end when I would drink to oblivion, eat like a star on *My 600-lb Life*, and refuse to do anything truly productive to make myself, my career, or my family Life better. I was still working in the legal field, though I knew that I was not where I needed to be. I was working myself to the bone in all the jobs for reasons unbeknownst to me, ignoring my kids in ways that I did not mean to do, and struggling to care about relationships that were supposed to matter. I believe this is called a lack of presence.

Summary: My "balanced" Life was living me—I was not living Life.

"We don't know how you do what you do," people would say to me.

I wanted to respond, "Beats me. I am pretty tired. And hungover. With a touch of suicidal." (And trust me, I do not say that lightly.) The entire time I was working on having it all, I felt a suicidal undertone to my inner being. I did not actually realize this was happening at the time. I wanted someone to tell me the way, the path; I wanted someone who was busy like me to tell me how to do it *better than me.*

If I ever showed the I-am-sort-of-teetering-on-the-edge cards to anyone (which I would sometimes do to strangers—usually when drinking—not my greatest attribute), then I would hear almost the same thing every single time: "Oh, dear, Meredith. You simply need balance." And they would say it like this: *bah-lance.*

I did not feel that I needed balance in my Life. I sensed that I needed to be who I was. I sensed that I was living someone else's Life, not my own, and that was the issue. That everyone else was telling me to be balanced—when I just needed to figure out what I wanted.

First, I wasn't always sure who I was.

Second, I didn't have the insight to make that decision to step into who I was (again, maybe because I didn't know who I was). Third, well, I was pretty much drinking all the time—and with that sort of numbing mechanism, you simply run out of cares to give.

Here's the truth about balance. Balance has the appearance of calm and wonder, but balance is complacency. Balance is stagnant. Balance is doing everything half-ass—making everyone else happy. It's synonymous with mediocre, where Dreams and aspirations go to die. To go after the Life you want, you cannot throw yourself in front of the balance train. It will surely kill you.

Back when the kids were young and I was "balancing" it all,* I remember the feeling of drowning. I remember thinking, I don't know how to make my Life better. I remember having repeated moments of not wanting to Live—it was all too hard and I was just so very tired.

We are often totally full of our own excuses and standing in our own way. But we are still hurting; we are still tired. We can suffer no matter what our Life presents. Comparing the modes of suffering between individuals is the worst thing you can do for yourself. Someone, somewhere abso-freaking-lutely has it harder and worse than you. But that's not the point. We are suffering.

And our suffering comes mostly from *our expectations.*[4]

"Folks who thrive in God's grace give grace easily, but the self-critical person becomes others-critical. We 'love' people the way we 'love' ourselves, and if we are not good enough, then no one is. . . . When we impose unrealistic expectations on ourselves, it's natural to force them on everyone else."[5]

Simply, we expect things to turn out a certain way—when our expectations crash disappointingly into our reality—suffering occurs.[6] We are further suffering because we find ourselves on a quest for balance. We expect balance to be the answer. We are told that balance is what we need. To work hard, be grateful, be everything to everyone, and then it will all be okay.

Then, when we fail to achieve this mystical balance because we are exhausted, impossibly drained, and not taking care of ourselves (because we can't possibly!), we suffer.

Because we can't make it all happen—something has to give for something else to be amazing. We certainly can't make everything

---

* My definition of balance back then was working a job I hated, allowing other people to raise my children, and doing ALL the things for everyone else to look like I had it together. The quest for balance was making me tired, miserable, a bad mother, and unhealthy. If you're a working mom and struggling with the balance phenomenon, read *Drop the Ball* by Tiffany Dufu.

look easy. And therefore, we are back to the original-sin lies: I will
never . . . I am always . . .

More on suffering in Chapter 5, but for now, recognizing the lie
of balance for what it is worth (an impossibility) will prove to be one
of the most valuable, freeing exercises you will encounter.

· · · · Checkpoint 3 ·

1. Name two of the most impactful lies you have
    been told by Other People. Have you been able
    to dismiss these lies, or have they become a part
    of your Core Beliefs?

2. Now, rewrite those lies.

Example:
> Lie: You will never be a runner.
> Rewrite: I *am* a runner.
> Lie: You will never find someone to love you.
> Rewrite: I am worthy of love.

3. How are you *suffering* right now? Be honest with
    yourself. We will come back to this, but write
    down your initial thoughts now: How are you
    suffering?

#RewriteTheLies #NoMoreLies #ISpeakTruth
#YearOfNoNonsense

4

Breaking Up with the Lies We Tell Ourselves

WHEN WE HAVE BEEN LIED TO OR MANIPULATED, WE CAN EASILY continue those same lies—or create fancy new ones to tell ourselves. So, we can totally tell Lies 1 to 3 in the previous chapter to ourselves, and those lies become part of our story, our inner workings, our Core Beliefs.

I sometimes tell myself that if I skip a workout, it won't matter. That ten pieces of pizza is fine. Of course, skipping workouts and pizza are objectively fine (we aren't food or workout shaming around here). But for me both can lead to incredibly destructive emotional and physical streaks—because I have issues with gluten and dairy, binge eating and perfectionism, self-loathing and addiction (to name a few). I lie to myself, then I suffer, then I hate myself for doing it, then I repeat the cycle because I just feel terrible physically and emotionally. I am causing my own suffering—on repeat. I know by now that workouts are key to my emotional Health and that overeating anything turns on my eat-all-the-things button and launches that cycle into orbit.

The "small" lies we tell ourselves can easily become a vicious and destructive series of events where we perpetuate the lies and then proceed to hate ourselves. Many of us don't even realize this cycle is happening. But once we open our eyes to the lies—all kinds—from all the people, including ourselves, then we can figure out what is Truth and how to move forward.

"You must keep the promises you make to yourself, and reward yourself, so that you can trust and motivate yourself," Jordan B. Peterson writes in *12 Rules for Life*.[1] Trusting ourselves is a new world for many of us. But it starts now.

LIE #4: I HAVE NO CHOICE

We make about 35,000 choices a day.[2] Apparently, we make over two hundred decisions each day around food alone. (I feel like I make about 20,000 decisions a day based on food.)[3]

When I was working in law and drowning in debt, I firmly believed I had no choice but to keep up the grind. To deal with said grind, I shoved a blueberry scone and a latte in my face every morning on the way to work. Some days I swore that the scone was the only thing keeping me alive. I could eat the scone, listen to the radio, and then work a full day. Eventually, when I started working out in the morning, I replaced the scone with training—and my body thanked me for that. But then I would eat a bagel with cream cheese after the workout—the bagel was just another form of a scone. I was missing the point, as I often do with food. Hence, 20,000 choices.

Irrespective of the bagel or scone, I was convinced that no other choices existed with regard to my profession. That in order to get out from under the mountain of debt, to take care of my family, and to make all my people proud, I was *required* to practice law, to make more money, to keep up with the Hustle.

But that wasn't about me; it was about my perception of Other People's expectations, and the script (remember that?), and my people-pleasing tendencies. More on people pleasing later.

CH-CH-CH-CHOICES

What do you feel like you have no choice in? Your job? Your X? Your Y? Here's my list from not so long ago:

> "But I have no choice to be an attorney. I went to freaking law school."
> "But I have no choice but to do triathlon. I am freaking *Swim Bike Mom*."
> "But I have no choice to be overweight and miserable. I have always been." (Ah-hem, see Lie #1, last chapter.)

As you can imagine, a Life of accepting these lies often points to all the lies being related and combining into one giant document: the script. The eradication of people pleasing comes with accepting that we want something different—and that we have a choice to decide to make that happen.

We have a choice between most components of our day. The choice might not be between Best Option Ever and Second-Best Option Ever—but a moment of decision and choice exists in most every situation.

- Wake up or hit snooze
- Shower or be stinky
- Coffee or no coffee. Creamer or no creamer; heavy cream, milk, coconut milk, or almond milk. Sugar or black or stevia or artificial chemicals. Big mug or small mug. Plastic or ceramic cup.

We have choice in much of our day. But we get into trouble when we try to control that which cannot be controlled: planes, trains, and automobiles, animals, weather, the news, and Other People and their decisions, actions, and consequences.

Summary: We spend time trying to control that which is outside our control and blaming everyone else for the things within our control.

Ouch.

Notwithstanding how I feel about princess tales and "holding out for the hero" garbage, I do love the story of the Princess and the pea:

> Once there was a Prince who wanted to marry a Princess. Only a real one would do. . . . One evening a terrible storm blew up. . . . Who should be standing outside but a Princess, and what a sight she was in all that rain and wind. . . . Yet she claimed to be a real Princess.
>
> . . . Without saying a word [the Queen] went to the bed-chamber, stripped back the bedclothes, and put just one pea in the bottom of the bed. Then she took twenty mattresses [and more] and piled them on the pea. . . . Up on top of all these the Princess was to spend the night.
>
> In the morning they asked her, "Did you sleep well?"
>
> "Oh!" said the Princess. "No. . . . I lay on something so hard that I'm black and blue all over. It was simply terrible."
>
> They could see she was a real Princess. . . . Nobody but a Princess could be so delicate. So the Prince made haste to marry her, because he knew he had found a real Princess.[4]

Aside from the fact that princess tales are a nightmare, I was less irked by the sexist outcome than by the princess's inaction.

As a little girl, I recall thinking, "She should have just slept on the couch."

What I took away from that tale—even ages ago—was that the Princess surely had many more choices than the freaky mattress tower. What about the floor? Another room? A table? The stable? Pull the mattresses down? Or hell, just get warm and get the hell out of there.

The point being—we always have choices. Sometimes they are as obvious as the ridiculousness of a mattress tower. We just aren't thinking about choice. We aren't approaching each moment with *what is my choice here?* Somehow, we are on stuck-in-rut autopilot.

Either that, or we see too many hard choices and become paralyzed—the consequences of all the choices fester in our brains. We look at them, we weigh them, we Fear them, we repeat—and then we stop. Deer in the headlights. We don't or can't or won't make a choice. The choices are too scary, too painful, or too risky. The Fear is real. The pain is real. The risk is real. The result is that nothing changes. We continue the cycle of absolutely nothing changing.

Regardless of whether we are ignoring the fact that we have choices or we are stuck in overanalysis, it's important to remember that we almost always have a choice.

LIE #5: JUST LOVE YOURSELF

Tess Holliday, a three-hundred-pound supermodel, hit the cover of *Cosmopolitan* in 2018. The public response to the cover swung wildly from "Finally!" and "Thank you, Cosmo" to "How dare you promote this fatness!" to "Oh my God, what if I *catch* that shit?"

When she was questioned about whether she was purposefully promoting an unhealthy lifestyle, Holliday's comment was solid gold:

> I can't even entertain [that question] respectfully. I'm not putting myself on the cover and saying, "Hey guys, let's all gain 300lbs and be fat." I'm literally just existing in my body. I don't

have to prove that I'm healthy to anybody. I'm so incredibly grateful to be able to exist in this space that people haven't been able to before. My health is no one's business. My message isn't, "Let's all be fat!" My message is, "Let's love yourself, regardless of how you look in your current body." Your mental health is far more important before you can worry about your physical health.[5]

This. Holy mother—so much this.

But I (still) struggle with the concept of "self-love" as a cure-all for what's going on in our Lives.

"Should" we love ourselves? Sure! That's a great thing.

But, I also argue that we simply can't wake up and begin to love ourselves—like *boom*—when self-loathing, disgust, and self-hate have been the norm. We can't just start loving. Some of us don't even know what love is, because our past examples of love (parents, siblings, relationships) are so messed up. We were treated poorly or inappropriately by those who "loved" us—and we think *that* is love. So self-love looks a lot like deprecating comments, cruel nicknames, inappropriate comments, and self-hate.

Some of us are incapable of simply waking up and starting with self-love because we have decades and decades of dislike for ourselves. Some of us have many, many more hurdles to leap over before we can even dip our toe in the sea of miraculous self-love.

Why? Because we have been living a Life of self-destruction or self-flagellation. How can we just instantly *love*?

Yes, we should have a good self-care practice. We should "love ourselves" enough not to feed our bodies trash, drown our gullets in vodka, or slice our inner thighs to release pain. We should care about our careers and fulfillment in Life and relationships. We shouldn't take Oxy or snort coke. We should not starve or gorge ourselves. We should not exercise out the meal we just ate or flush it down the toilet by way of vomit or laxatives. We should practice yoga, meditate, and breathe in the cool fucking moonlight.*

I know. Self-care is super.

But some of us have been drowned, beaten, and cracked wide open by the body-image conundrum, by abuse, rape, and other heinous circumstances. We have been made to believe that we had the perfect childhood or marriage only to discover later, in a flash, that it was all a lie. We can't open up and begin to love and care for ourselves when our foundation upon which many of our beliefs have been built upon suddenly crumbles. In cases of abuse (actual or covert), our bodies might be scary. Our souls feel broken. We don't even want to be in the body we have, let alone love on it.

Self-love? What is that? There's just too much there to overcome for some of us right now. So you won't hear me say, "Love yourself" or "Practice self-care."

But you will hear me say, "Clear out the Nonsense in your Life."

Not even Nonsense about your body or your hair. Just the general Nonsense in day-to-day Life. Nonsense straight from the opening list on page xi. What on that list can you eradicate?

With less of the practical Nonsense comes space and air—breath and some light. In that cleared space, we can begin to see that self-love and self-care are possible actions. We peel the Truth Onion and keep peeling. We may not be ready to go there yet, but with each day, we can envision a time and a place where we might be ready.

In our Pursuit of Happiness, we see small places where self-love and self-care might begin to grow. Little by little, we can do a few nice

---

* Use of the word "should" here is somewhat snarky but also true. Telling someone what they should and should not do is not my jam. "Should," in this context, is meant to be considered from a general place of wellness and lining up with the theme of decent self-care behaviors.

things for ourselves: read a book, buy some nice slippers (not glass, of course), or put some fresh paint on the walls in a room in our home.

Meeting ourselves where we *are* is a fundamental tool of self-love and growth. Acceptance of ourselves is important, but so is the capability to grow and change. No one has proved the hypothesis to me that we must accept where we are, right here and right now. I hear that touted (first is acceptance), but I don't buy it. Sometimes we have to change in a way or two before we can accept. There's nothing wrong with taking that path either.

To me, the first step toward self-love and self-care is seeing the Truth.

We must see where we are right now. We must open our eyes and see the sights and Truth about where we are and what is going on in our Lives. But then, we can accept or absolutely reject it. But in order to even reject, we must see the Truth. If we reject, then we obviously want to change. So, moving beyond our circumstances or bullshit is the next step, along with tapping into our Resources. Finally, leaping into our Purpose—or rather, Living Life on your terms, right now—is the final rung. Maybe that involves your body; maybe it doesn't.

Society lies to us.

But we also lie to ourselves about what reality is and what a strong and healthy version of ourselves—physically and emotionally—is. Loving ourselves and caring for ourselves is fundamental, but we can't always just start immediately. We may need to start with the Truth and go from there.

The simplest need, truly, is compassion for ourselves. We are on a quest and a journey—and we need to understand that the act of *seeing* is hard. And it's okay to want more, to work for more, and to do what makes you feel *good*. Exploring this topic is beyond the scope of this book, but keep going and doing the work—it is a big key to cracking through some Nonsense.

···· Checkpoint 4 ···

1. Name two lies you have been telling yourself. Why do you believe you continue to tell yourself these lies? What needs do these lies fulfill?

2. Rewrite those lies.
   > Lie: I will always be stuck in this job.
   > Rewrite: I have a choice, and I can choose to create a new path.

#RewriteTheLies #NoMoreLies #ISpeakTruth #YearOfNoNonsense

PART II

THRIVE IN THE PRESENT

- Welcome to the Truth Onion
- About the Other People
- About That Hustle and Grit
- About Those Hopes and Dreams
- Social Media—How to Deal
- Setting Boundaries
- Getting Rid of Toxic People and Things
- You Are Resourceful

5

Peeling the Truth Onion

TRY WRITING A BOOK ABOUT NONSENSE WHEN YOU'VE JUST EATEN four bowls of cereal after dinner. Stupid. I struggle with binge eating but not purging. The Lifelong battle between the food I "should"* feed my body and the food I want to eat is real. But regardless of what I eat, I don't purge. I just go straight from the binge to the self-hate. My purge is the self-hate. If you don't think that's bad, then let's explore a recent conversation with my husband.

"I ate so much tonight," I said.

"Come on. What did you actually eat? It's not like you had an entire bucket of chicken."

I didn't say anything. He looked at me.

"You didn't eat a bucket of chicken, did you?"

"No," I said, "but I had an entire bag of Goldfish crackers."

"That's okay. What else?"

"Chocolate."

---

* Again, use of the word "should" is snarky.

"And?"

"Chips. The waffle kettle ones—"

"And?"

This next part was the part I knew would sink the ship.

"Lasagna. Out of the trash."

"Oh, Mere," he said, wide-eyed.

Then I laughed. Because what else could I do? I had just admitted to my husband of almost seventeen years that I am a Trash Panda Dumpster Diver—a TPDD.

He knew exactly what lasagna I was talking about too. He had asked me after dinner, "Do you want this last piece of veggie lasagna before I toss it?"

Knowing that pasta and tomatoes and cheese are my kryptonite, I said, "No, just toss it." I had eaten a lovely salmon salad. I was proud of myself. Then the family left for a movie. I didn't go directly for the trash. That came after the Goldfish and chocolate and chips.

But then, I did. I went for the trash. I knew the lasagna was wrapped in foil. It was still warm. *What's a girl to do?*

Well, a girl who doesn't have a binge-eating problem probably leaves the trash lasagna in the trash. But I ate it, and it was good. I mean, it was amazing. And I'm technically not one bit sorry about it. So. There you go. My name is Meredith, I am writing about finding and getting rid of Nonsense, and I eat out of the trash.

But my TPDD raiding tendencies are my reality. That's what I did, and I'm telling you now. Because it's true. Because my eating habits can sometimes be trash and Nonsense, and I have to work at them every day—every single day.

Yes, we've been lied to. Yes, we've been lying to ourselves. When we are faced with these lies, we have a choice to make: we can get mad and tell the Truth (and then do something), or we can stick our heads in the sand and pretend we didn't just eat out of the trash (and therefore do nothing about this problem). Or, worse—we feel deep and dark shame about eating out of the trash—so we hide and shame ourselves. At least admitting the trash eating? I no longer have shame about it.

You can feel any range of emotion at the lies. Anger need not necessarily be the "correct" emotion. However, by disallowing the feelings or hiding them, numbing them with whatever mechanism, we give the problems teeth. Sticking our heads in the sand is not the way to go. Nothing to see but lies down in the sand.

(Did you know that sand is actually *made* of 99.9 percent lies? True story.)

If you keep your head out of the sand, then you are able to see and feel what is happening. You can observe the lies. You can confront the context. With heads up and clarity, you can take action to stop perpetuating an internal and external culture of abuse and shame. With your eyes open, you find courage and bravery to do what you *must*. Sure, you have experienced a Lifetime of lies told by others. But how often has your inner voice then taken up the flag and screamed those lies on repeat?

You can easily feel stuck and permanently mired in the quicksand of your own making.

(You might feel like you want to freak out.)

Maybe it is time to freak out. I mean, you've been lied to (and worse). You've also been perpetuating these lies or creating more of them to cover up the other ones in order to make Life make sense. You now know that Nonsense abounds. Much of what you thought was true is clearly Nonsense. You aren't doing what you want to do with your Life. Balance is bullshit! So is Happiness! Everything is a mess!

Truth.

Life is messy.

Dr. Brené Brown talks about her "vulnerability hangover" after giving a TED talk in Houston.[1] She publicly told a large group of people that she, a researcher in shame and vulnerability, had experienced a breakdown. She'd had a breakdown because all the years of research she had conducted gave her answers that she did not want. The great body of work she conducted revealed a Truth that she was not ready for.

As a result of this "breakdown," however, Dr. Brown has become one of the most incredible self-help icons of our time. She has taught us that vulnerability is our most accurate measurement of courage, that by being who we are, the most authentic versions of ourselves, we have the power to innovate, create, and change—not only ourselves but the world around us.

A similar thing happened to me when I understood that I was budding with Nonsense: a Nonsense Hangover.

That's the path. Truth, then pain and work, and then a sense of lightness, hope, and freedom. But a path is still a somewhat uncharted road—and sometimes we don't have a clear route in place to begin to work through all our hurts, feelings, and pain. The Year of No Nonsense is just this path—a sometimes slippery, trash lasagna path.

But on the upside, the path is well lit and marked with clues . . . and it has been traveled.

REALITY IS (TAKE A DEEP BREATH)

I have some more bad news. To get rid of Nonsense, you must have a realistic picture of your current, sometimes terrible and dark state of affairs. (Might sound a little like emotional intelligence and self-awareness.) In other words, we need to see. (Yes. Seeing. The dead horse of the book—we need to see. But seeing is very, very important.)

In group yoga classes, a teacher may begin by asking the class participants to notice where they are. I love how they say, "Take notice of how you have arrived on your mat," like I was beamed there. Let me tell you how I arrived on this mat, I think in a huff. (Exactly. I am someone who needs more yoga in her Life.) Without judgment, without much comment, the instructor may urge us to make a short assessment of how we feel sitting on our respective mats. What aches in our bodies?

What is our mind doing? Are we angry or sad? In about one minute, a person who is sitting still might actually recognize exactly how he or she is feeling.

Which is often why I run out of yoga like my ass is on fire. Turns out you can't force me to sit still with my own thoughts for long. I also don't like actually being in this body I inhabit. Like my psychotherapist friend Britt Frank says, "I am a floating head." Totally. Working to grow into a contemplative, calm, and meditative person who sits in her own body comfortably is literally the hardest work I have ever done.

But I do meditate now. I also meditate while working out without even realizing it—it's called *moving meditation*. Moving my body in hard and deliberate ways *is* a form of body awareness and mindfulness that resonates most with me. When I finish workouts, I often hardly remember being there.

Meeting yourself (seeing) where you are is necessary.

Meeting yourself (seeing) without judgment is hard but also necessary.

There is a stark difference between meeting yourself (seeing) where you are and accepting everything, your Life, and your circumstances *forever* where you currently are. No one says you can't change or take a different path. But in order to change anything, you do have to know where you *are*. Again, we must see.

We can make meditation and mindfulness whatever we want.*
The moral of the mediation story? You need not do anything that doesn't feel organic to you. We've spent our whole lives trying to *do* and *be* things that aren't necessarily us. The fact that we need not sit or

---

* Noting that meditation, mindfulness, and manifestation can be considered separate practices, I am using the general term "meditation" here as I am not trained (or overly skilled) in any of the three. For example, qigong and tai chi, walking or standing meditation, and, my new favorite, daily Life practice meditation—where you essentially reduce the speed of everyday activities and use the extra time to practice mindfulness and focus on thoughts—are all types of outside-the-box meditation. Daily Life practice meditation is one of the ways I tackle my laundry—if I tackle it at all.

be still was a game changer that opened the door to meditation. Now I can (and do) sit still, too.

Meditation aside, an important part of the Year of No Nonsense process is a Self-Inventory of your Life's contents (coming up in Part III). In an inventory, with the same acceptance practiced in a yoga class, you are recognizing what is (and is not) and making an honest assessment. You're counting what you have in your Life, in yourself, and the things you don't—not in an ungrateful way, just in an observatory manner. You are assessing the Truth of the matter(s) in your Life and putting the Names, Numbers, and figures into a hypothetical spreadsheet in a way that doesn't hurt or harm you. Merely, objective observation. So you know what's up.

Imagine if an Amazon warehouse decided to both take and rearrange all its inventory at once. Everything has a department, then a subdepartment, and then even more categories—and for good reason. That's why you can't find a proper spatula in a search for "books" on Amazon. (Though you will turn up a book called *The Spatula*.)

All parts of us, likewise, require a proper place, space, and context. We need to figure out what parts of us and our lives are what (and what is not truly us). We need an inventory process. Therefore, we begin with the Truth.

WHAT IS TRUE

We've established that our Life is likely full of Lies and Nonsense. Yay us.

So how can we make an accurate inventory of our lives when all the Numbers, Names, data, boxes, and labels are wrong? That's a fair question. So we must discern the Truth about ourselves. We must understand the lies.

Byron Katie's work revolves around just that.

She teaches a self-inquiry method known as "The Work." The Work didn't get that Name out of nowhere. The Work is *hard work*. The Work is also simple and described as "a way to identify and question the thoughts that cause all of your *suffering*."[2]

Truth and suffering are related.

Suffering is a true thing.

Therefore, in order to get to Truth, we need to talk about suffering in more depth. (You thought we could be done with that, didn't you?)

SUFFERING: LEARNING TO FEEL

My suicide attempt was about suffering.

I was twenty years old. I was prescribed Zoloft "for my depression," and I was ballooning up in weight. At 240, I just kept eating and stopped weighing.

The most memorable binge meal was two Whopper cheeseburgers, two large fries, two orders of cheese sticks, and a half order of jalapeno poppers (I ate half only because they were just too spicy). Then I had ice cream. I have always eaten a lot, but during that period, I was binging beyond all space and time and reason. I drank daily—copious amounts of booze. I pushed people away completely. I cared only about drinking and eating and watching a weird soap opera called *Passions*—that was literally so terrible, I can't believe I am admitting it. It's worse than eating out of the trash. I stayed inside, drunk, bloated, hidden, embarrassed by my body and my habits.

The Truth?

At twenty years old, I had given up Hope of a good Life. Worst of all, I didn't know why (at the time). I just knew I had given up.

Life was dark.

One night, I mixed my regularly scheduled Zoloft with a whole lot of vodka and cigarettes. I called my boyfriend and told him I was going to kill myself. I sat on the front porch and sawed superficial cuts into my left arm, waiting for him to arrive. When he showed up, he took the dull knife from me. I told him I was going to slice my wrists, and he said, "No, you aren't."

We were standing in the kitchen. In one movement, I opened a drawer, grabbed another knife, raised my arms, and sliced downward, hard.

I *showed* him.

He grabbed a dish towel and held my wrist so tight that he hurt me. My roommate called 911. I was carted off to the hospital, where I had a blood alcohol content of .36—which is the amount of alcohol for most people to be in a coma, if not dead.

I remember a few things from the following twenty-four hours: the ambulance ride and praying that I wouldn't die. And hoping the cops didn't find my fake ID. Calling my mom, telling her I tried to kill myself, and her screaming, then throwing the phone onto what sounded like the floor. *Hello? Mom?* The three days that I had to go to a treatment center—where they placed me with the psychiatric patients instead of the substance abuse folks. That I smelled like some combo of booze, wet dog (not sure why), and onions for two days.

I remember that the center let me go home with no follow-up. I just left and was sent out into the wide world. Maybe because I was good at playing the game.

I don't remember all that happened on that night because I—the real me—was not present. I was numbed by antidepressants. I was high on vodka. I was a mess from all the sugar and chemical foods I was eating and the lack of exercise and—also—sunlight. I had locked myself inside the apartment for the most part, aside from classes, shutting myself away from the world.

My decline from a "normal"* student to a drunk, depressed, and suicidal recluse was not a long process either. I went from mildly sad to sliced wrist in three months. Three months was all it took from me telling a doctor that I was "depressed" to almost losing my Life by my own hand.

It's easier to say that I didn't want to die and I wasn't there that night. It makes the whole incident somehow more forgivable, less "shameful." I always say that it wasn't "me" that day—it was Zoloft and vodka, sugar and sadness, hopelessness and shame.

But the Truth of the matter is that sometimes those things *are* me: sugar and sadness, hopelessness and shame. So it *was* me. I was there. So much hopelessness, shame.

Dr. Brown writes, "Shame is lethal . . . shame is deadly. And I think we are swimming in it deep. Shame needs three things to grow exponentially in our lives: secrecy, silence, and judgment."[3]

Here's the bottom line: "Shame cannot survive being spoken," Brown says. "It cannot survive empathy."

So I spoke and continue to speak: nearly two decades later, before I quit drinking for good, I would think about driving myself into a tree. This giant tree at the bottom of a hill on a road I drove often. I was *sugar and sadness, hopelessness and shame.* I was working out all the time but miserable and unhealthy. It was just varying degrees. It was controlled Whopper and vodka consumption, socially acceptable decay by destruction. I had improved my Life, but for the most part, I thought I might just drive into the tree and be done with all the feelings, the suffering.

I drank so I felt nothing. I ate so I felt nothing. I shopped online so I felt nothing. I created massive diversions like redecorating, throwing myself into new projects that I didn't have time for. Feelings—

---

* I have been some version of depressed, sad, and suicidal for as long as I can remember. It just all came to a head with this behavior. So "normal" was never good. And what is normal anyway?

and feeling my body—were the things that hurt the most. I am a floating head.

Getting sober became about force-feeling the feelings of my Life. Feeling my feelings turned out to be the hardest thing that I have ever had to do up until that time. (Now feeling my feelings in my body and not as a floating head is that same pain.)

Miraculously, though, since being sober, I have not thought about ending my Life. I have learned to understand and feel the feelings and not turn to booze to wash the feelings away or to shame them. Recovery from addiction, suffering, or mental illness is not easy or seamless, I know that. But there is Hope and power—we have it inside us.

First, we must start with understanding that we are suffering, and we don't need to be suffering. We must see, and we must see that.

If you don't feel right in your mind or body, then something isn't right. If you are depressed, I understand. Take a look at your habits, your Life, your childhood. Where does the suffering come from? Take a look at your medication. Did your Life get worse or better with it? Are you mixing it with a cocktail? Make sure you have a doctor or therapist who is trauma-informed and who listens to and sees and treats you as a whole person, and not a floating head.

Before we lose Hope, we must remove the barriers (Nonsense) from our Lives that are impeding the ability for the light to shine in. We must remove those things that are literally roadblocking any chance we might have to Live our best Life. Whether it's booze or food or the wrong prescription, the wrong people or job, or even the wrong family members, taking a moment to question what might be driving the pain, the sadness, and the suffering can be eye-opening.

Not to trivialize anyone's suffering, but oftentimes our suffering is connected directly to Nonsense, our own or someone else's.

Our aversion to feeling pain and sadness is understandable. Who wants to feel hurt and sadness? It's much easier to dodge the anguish and replace those feelings with the addiction or diversion du jour. The cycle of pain doesn't end with the numbing, though. The cycle digs itself a deeper hold—diversion, numbing, and then shame. Shame—on a repeated cycle—morphs into hopeless. And that feeling of hopeless is what drives us beyond the perceived ability to repair, beyond reason, and toward thinking Life is, or should be, over. We must address our suffering before we reach hopeless.

Suffering, as mentioned before, may be the result of our unmet expectations. When what we expect out of Life is drastically different from what Life gives or takes, and we don't have the proper tools or awareness to deal with the Truth, the feelings, and the result, then the spiral can begin. We don't want the feelings, so we numb. With the numbing comes the hopeless-shame cycle.

Many people are uneasy with the idea that their Lives contain suffering. They want to believe that suffering does not rise to the level of "true" suffering unless it's "huge"—but that's part of the problem. The word itself—suffering—gives us pause.

Often we think, "Oh, but this person has it so much worse than I do." We close ourselves off. We isolate ourselves. We feel that our suffering is not worthy of discussing, so we go off into a corner to suffer further by ourselves while thinking, This isn't suffering.

But Truth time.

When we expect Life, love, profession, self, and reality to be a certain way (aka "Happiness"), and we find ourselves in a completely opposite world, we suffer. We hear from the outside world, "You should be grateful" and "#blessed." And that might be true. But we can suffer immensely—no matter what the reality is. Then we hear various forms of comparison as to why our suffering is not real, or gratitude and meditation will solve it. Of course we should be grateful and meditation is great, but if we feel suffering, then we are suffering. We have to work to not suffer—that may be our current Truth. See it. Don't look away.

Why are we ranking problems or suffering on any sort of scale? We should be thinking about why *we are suffering* in the first place. Do not ask the question, "Should I be allowed to suffer, when Sally has it so much worse?" Remove that comparison from your thoughts, because you need to get to the reason why you (not Sally) are suffering. "*Suffering* comes from a Latin word *ferre*, which translates as 'to bear' or 'to carry.' . . . When you deny or resist the experience of your own suffering, you are unwilling to consciously bear it. It is this resistance to accepting your Life just as it is that makes suffering feel ignoble, despicable, and shameful."[4]

Those are three impressive synonyms for suffering: *ignoble, despicable, shameful*. But consider it for a minute. How many times have we struggled with something that tore our insides to shreds, but we felt unentitled to feel that way? *Ignoble. Despicable. Shameful.* Pretty accurate.

I went through a period in my Life when I had a steady stream of internal suffering—for reasons I couldn't identify or articulate. But looking back, I can now identify "resistance to accepting my Life," as articulated above. Additionally, I had some unresolved trauma that I had not yet begun to explore. At the time, though, I felt that something was *wrong* with me. So, since I was in need of "fixing," I would go to a doctor or a psychiatrist and leave with a prescription, thinking, "Okay, I will be fixed now."

I trusted someone else to fix me—and that was where I went wrong. I did not trust myself. I never had.

I learned that I had to fix me. I had to ask the right questions, keep digging. Professionals could help and guide me (and therapy is a great idea for many), but it is not the job of a professional to fix me—it was my job to do the work.

Or . . . maybe I didn't actually need fixing. Because I wasn't broken. I was just a little rough, a little cracked, a little more floating head than present in my body.

Maybe I just had some hard work to do.

It's the same for all of us: nothing is "wrong" with us. We are suffering, and we need to recognize and understand those feelings in order to get through it, to actually learn how to fix the suffering—once and for all. Again, we don't necessarily need to relive any traumatic or past experiences. Rather, we just need to recognize that these things happened and work to move past these issues.

I believed that I needed fixing because, well, I was suffering. Because I was suffering, I believed I was broken. If I (or someone else) fixed me, then the suffering would stop. If a doctor told me what was wrong with me and prescribed a pill, then I would be fixed.

We are the cause of our continued suffering. However, it's not because we are broken, and the origin may not be our fault. But we *are* perpetuating Nonsense, which is leading to our additional and continued suffering about the same things—for years and years. The extra Nonsense might be what is continuing the suffering that was started elsewhere by someone else.

We are responsible for our healing. So we need a little Truth, a plan, and less Nonsense, in order to work toward our best Life. That will lead to less suffering.

Once I opened my eyes to what Truth and lies abounded in my Life, I found other ways to deal with some of my anxiety, stress, Fear, and "bipolar"-isms. For example, once when I was told I was bipolar, I accepted a bipolar diagnosis. What I ignored, though, was the small fact that I was also throwing down booze every night to make myself most certainly an alcohol-induced bipolar. I came down at night with booze, and I was thrust up into a crazy world in the morning when I woke up. I felt bipolar, yep. Who wouldn't? But did that *make* me bipolar?

I also accepted a diagnosis of irritable bowel syndrome and diverticulitis after two powerful incidents that sent me to the ER. Followed by a severe bout of shingles—where I looked like Sloth from *The Goonies* for a span of ten days.

As I look back to the times when I had all these "Health"—physical and mental—problems, my day was this:

5 a.m.: Wake and work out (after going to bed at midnight, drunk)

7 a.m.: Get kids to school, then sit in traffic with giant latte and sugary scone

8 a.m.: Work at desk all damn day

1 p.m.: Order in some sort of brown food to the office

4 p.m.: Sit in traffic with another giant latte

5 p.m.: Pick up kids from after-school care (bitter and cranky kids who had eaten a sugary, establishment-provided snack)

6 p.m.: Pour a glass of wine

7 p.m.: Dinner with wine

8 p.m.: Kids to bed with wine (me, not them)

9 p.m.: Wine and eat until midnight bedtime (and fight with my husband at some point)

I followed this exact schedule, more or less, for nearly a decade. Before kids, I had a similar schedule, leaving out the kid duties. Before triathlon, I did the same thing—just without the wake and work out component. But the lack of sleep, the drinking, and the brown food? Well, that remained the same for nearly two decades. Naturally, the culmination of these years might result in someone developing diverticulitis, shingles, and bipolar disorder. Those are symptoms, too, of me not dealing with some real stuff from the past: trauma, shame, and more.

I know now that I was (am) not alone.

Hordes of us are doing these destructive things, juxtaposed with random "healthy" things like working out—on the daily—and wondering why we are depressed, miserable, lost. I also know that what works for my Health doesn't necessarily work for everyone, but I do believe that the *process* works for all of us. Again, we are doing these destructive things for a *reason*. We do not want to feel the pain of the past, the shame of the present, Fear of the future, or whatever other emotions we continue to dodge.

Truth is not revealed overnight.

Truth is an onion.

The Truth Onion is a real thing.

When we decide to look at our Truth, we are tapping into the crackly outer skin of the Truth Onion. But, the Truth Onion keeps on stinking and gets even stronger as you peel closer to its core.

Which is why we are perhaps unwilling to start peeling it at all.

I believed I had visited the core of my Truth Onion. But then, out of the blue, I peeled a *huge* layer about my past. And—a whole new Truth Onion appeared out of nowhere. I wasn't ready for it, and I thought: *Well, this changes my certainty about, I don't know—everything.*

I did not count on the fact that once I had peeled a Truth Onion, other freaking Truth Onions would appear. But that's how it goes. Your future is cloudy with a chance of more Truth Onions.

This new peeling has taken me straight to the place of my longest source of suffering—bam! As I write, I am currently in some pain (see, I told you—timely). But I know a few things: I will not always hurt just like this. And in order to stop this particular suffering, I must keep peeling to the Truth of this particular onion. Peeling is part of Life and part of Nonsense eradication.

Understanding that we are suffering is a place to start getting through this damn Truth Onion (and the ones that follow), even after we think we are done peeling. Understanding, too, that once we peel to what seems like the core—there still might be more to go. Life will always present us with more—and we can learn that we are strong enough to embrace each hard moment.

I am able, today, to tell myself: You are discovering this new layer at this time because you are now strong enough to handle it. Ten years ago, you would not have been. Keep going. Feel the pain. Know it won't last forever. Keep going . . .

MORE FROM THE TRUTH ONION

Byron Katie's "The Work" breaks down almost anything that comes across our paths into four simple questions, only two of which I will mention here.

The first question: Is it true? (Yes or no.)[5]

The next question, summarized: If it's not true, can you ever actually *learn* whether it is true or not? (In other words, is it an emotional response or something wholly factual, like "this tree exists.")

From those two questions Katie extends the exploration to our reactions about change—but you'll notice that she starts with Truth.

At the time I began the sport of triathlon, I had no idea what I was doing. I had no idea how to become a triathlete. I only knew that I was quite large, depressed, and angry. I knew that I couldn't stay where I was. Mind you, I didn't know where I was going—but it was the proverbial "closing time," and I had to find a new place to be. During this time, I learned that I enjoyed taking Spinning® classes. I didn't ask myself the question "Is it true" directly, but by moving my body, I intuitively found the answer to this question.

Is it true that I actually enjoy moving my body in a way that doesn't involve chips or margaritas or salsa—the food not the dance? *Holy hell*—it IS true! Maybe I might like to do some more moving.

My Spinning instructor told me about a year later, "You could do a triathlon if you wanted to." Again, I didn't know The Work at the time, but I wondered, "Is it true?"

The funny thing is that, after some doubting, I said, "Yes. Sure. Of course, I could. Why not?" and I went forward.

I perhaps could not do a first triathlon fast or fabulously, but the answer to "Is it true that I can do a triathlon?" was

Yes, this is true. Of course I can. Why not? Who says I can't?

I continued to apply this question to statements that I tried to declare as true.

- No one loves me. (Is it true? Yes or no.) No. *My kids love me. My lizard loves me.*
- I can never get out of the legal profession. (Is it true? Yes or no.) No. *I could quit right this second and leave. I am not a hostage.*
- I am so fat. (Is it true? Yes or no.) No. *I have fat; I am not fat.*

These questions made some real sense to me. I did "work" in the way of my Health and stress over the years. Like exiting a stressful and unfulfilling profession, and figuring out how to lovingly parent my children without losing my mind. To keep going and peeling the Truth Onion, I continue to ask the question *Is it true?* With this question, I am able to choose my *Names* and *Numbers* more carefully, purposefully. I think often about Truth, the lies, the things I am perpetuating—are these good or not so great?

By answering the question about Truth, we can see a path—a possible way out of our current suffering.

Translation: *Is this true? Hell no! It's Nonsense! So why in the world do I keep saying it!? That doesn't make sense! I can do better. I can say better things. This is a lie! This is not working for me. I am gonna change this. Starting right fresh now.*

The Work goes on to connect the power of beliefs, attitudes, and thoughts and is an amazing resource. Once we assess what is *true*, we place ourselves in the most powerful position: we can see clearly and begin to peel the stinky Truth Onion.

Remember the tree that I often thought of driving myself into? *I could drive myself into that giant pine tree and that would be it.* (If you know anything about pine trees, you know those aren't the bendy type of tree.) If someone had asked me during that time if I was suicidal, I would have said, "No! What do you mean?" In other words, I would have lied right through my teeth. I may not have admitted that I was suicidal, but I wanted out of this Life, as evidenced by my thoughts.

I want to drive myself into that tree. (Is it true? Yes or no.)

The answer was most certainly no. I did not *want* to drive myself into the tree.

I just wanted out of *this Life that I had made*—not necessarily Life in general. I just wanted better, more fulfilling. I wanted different. I wanted more from myself. I knew I could be better and different and more, but I didn't know how. I had a case of "resistance to accepting my Life"—also known as . . . *suffering.*

There it is again.

With the Truth, we know certain things to be true: too much junk food is "bad," sleep is good, exercise is good, love is lovely. But those are surface-level, commonsense-type Truths. Where we get stuck is in the minutiae of ourselves or our pasts, in focusing on the concentration and difficulty (and pain) that it will take to peel the Truth Onion. We don't want to feel it, and maybe we aren't always ready. The layers are endless, stinky, and tough. How do we get beyond the first layer, let alone all the layers?

TRUE TRUTH

For those who are still with my vegetable analogies, the outer core is the toughest.

And you're still with me, so you've already begun the peeling believe it or not. But all that peeling is to get us somewhere—namely, the True Truth—the Truth Onion's *core.* We find Truth with each peel, but we make it to the Truth Onion core by digging deeper still.

When starting to peel, I begin with this question: *What are some of the positive things I feel to be true about myself?*

- I work hard.
- I love my family.
- I am driven and goal oriented.
- I am loyal (until I am not).

What are some of the negative things I feel to be true about myself and my Life? Not labels like *I am fat* but pertinent statements (with verbs) about habits or behaviors. Some things from my past:

- I can act impatient.
- I tend to drink too much.
- I have a messy relationship with food.
- I can get angry on a dime.
- I do not exercise because I feel embarrassed about my body.
- I do not exercise because I don't have the time.
- I fantasize about divorce because I feel unhappy in my marriage.
- I do not give my best effort at my job because I do not like this work.

The True Truth is that place of self-awareness and honesty where we understand things that just are—for what they are. The core, the center. The meeting of the self on the damn Life mat.

So back to the blessed Truth Onion. It looks like this. The surface of the Truth Onion says, "I don't exercise because I don't have time." *You peel a layer.*

"I don't exercise because I am tired." *Peel a layer.*

"I am tired because I drink too much at night." *Peel a layer.*

"I drink too much because I am unhappy in my marriage." *Keep peeling.*

"I am unhappy in my marriage because I think it is a prison." *Peel, mofo, peel! Dance, monkey, dance! Peel!*

"I think marriage is a prison because my parents trapped themselves in a marriage they hated." *Peel.*

"As a child, I watched them fight, and it scared me." *Peel more.*

"Marriage still scares me. I am scared." *Peeeeeel.*

"I have a Core Belief that I will end up in a marriage like my parents'. So I am making a mess of my own even though I want desperately to be happy in this marriage—with this person." *Holy cow.*

Maybe some time passes, and you realize there is more. Maybe . . . "It's not just my parents' marriage, I guess, that scared me. But my dad—actually—he scared me." *Peel.*

"I just felt like I was being watched, judged. I never felt safe in my home . . ."

" . . . or my body." *Peel.*

"I wondered constantly if I was in real, substantial danger . . . because of the way he looked at me, judged my body. Stared . . ."

And there it is—the big wound: "I never felt safe in my home, around my dad, or in my body." That process majorly sucked, but you peeled to it—as long as it took. You scraped off some Nonsense, peeled past even more Nonsense, straight to the True Truth core of it all. This wound touches right on the fact that you don't like to exercise—because you don't like to feel your body, and perhaps so much as you don't want to draw attention to it—because you don't feel safe in it. Wow, right?

And whether Freudian or Jungian or none of them, you may have a wound from the past that keeps causing your present and future trouble.

That's what you must continue to peel to. *Boom.* Onion core. *True Truth.*

By the time you get to the core of the Truth Onion, you've made an incredible list of more Truths—ones that get truer, scarier, and perhaps more painful the further you peel. But you have a framework for so many types of Nonsense that must be changed.

Admitting that you are embarrassed about your body and that's why you don't exercise in public is a great starting point. Once you stand in your True Truth, you can begin to strip away the blame, the excuses, and the other lies that stem from these issues. That you don't have to be fearful seven-year-olds at the pool anymore. Or creeped-out sixteen-year-olds. Or adults who had trauma they are just now uncovering. When you see the True Truth, you can see the path to changing the things you *must* change. You aren't stuck in that script.

When you get to the core of the Truth Onion, you can think about rebuilding your entire Life—so you can Live.

If you have your head in the sand, let's try to pull it out. No one likes to look at reality. But we must. The True Truth is a place of comfort, though. Once we know something about ourselves (I do not go to the gym because I am embarrassed about my body—not because I am lazy—and I am embarrassed about my body because *something* happened when I was a young girl—and this might have something to do with all of this [?!]), then we can do something about it. There is comfort in Truth, because there is a directional line to draw. Oh, this might have happened. The comfort will come in knowing the Truth, even if it doesn't appear right away.

How many of us have spent months, years, and (in my case) *decades* doing the same insane things and expecting different results? I drank for decades. I expected to have a healthy Life because I was doing tri-athlon and sort of eating well. By my calculations, I thought I should be able to eat "okay," work out a stupid number of hours, and then drink myself into a coma each night—and be fit and healthy. *Insanity.* I spent DECADES eating less-than-ideal foods and expecting to lose fat. *Insanity.*

I *knew* this behavior was insane. Yet I stuck my head in the sand and sought other alternatives and other mechanisms to blame for my current state (or states), or as I have realized recently—to escape my past, to not peel, to not feel.

Sarah Hepola, author of *Blackout: Remembering the Things I Drank to Forget*, put a description of this insanity in a podcast interview. Like me, Sarah was a blackout drinker. So in order to keep continuing to drink she made a bargain with herself to try yoga and every thirty-day detox challenge on the planet. When those didn't work, she was a failure.

But the True Truth? All she needed to do was quit drinking.

For me, in my drinking "prime," I would do all the triathlons in the world—including the long IRONMAN ones. I would blog and appear like I was doing great. I was falling apart and trying all the "healthy" things. But I truly needed to just quit drinking. Quitting drinking was the problem core of my Truth Onion at the time; since then I have peeled it even further. I drank to not feel, I thought. Now I know that I drank to not remember.

And that has changed my True Truth even more.

So, we create all these other distractions and "new changes" to avoid the True Truth about ourselves, our Lives.

This isn't a book about teetotaling—even if it might seem like it sometimes. But I talk about that because it's what I know, it's what I have overcome, and that has been the path to my Truth. Everyone has their own version of drinking—their own avoidance, numbing mechanism. The analogies work, no matter the venom.

WHAT IS YOUR BOOZE?

Maybe booze is your booze. Maybe peanut butter is. But most of us have a certain poison sticking to us, making us stuck—from addictions to habits to bad relationships to self-destructive tendencies—behaviors that we do for a reason. I knew that I needed to stop drinking. I didn't want to. I wanted to make a deal with the devil to continue my shitty way of pretending to be healthy and happy.

Why wasn't that possible? It just didn't seem fair.

Quitting drinking was just the start of it, unfortunately. There were more issues and changes ahead. I needed to get control over some other bad habits: binge eating, binge spending, binge watching, binge iPhone-ing. I had (have) a binge problem.

I had (have) a Nonsense problem. (We all do.)

However, I knew that if I started on *all the things* at once, I would turn around and quit. Because *who can change everything in their Life?*

The answer is: Me. You. We all can.

But do we want to? Are we *willing*? What then?

This question is bigger than the Truth.

Because we can get to the True Truth, see it, see the resulting impact and walk away from it. Deciding what to do with that True Truth intel? That's the tricky part.

Maybe we want to stay stuck because it's familiar, it's what we know. Change is scary, the outcome unknown. (If we peel back the layers, who knows what we will find?!) If we repeat the same garbage habits over and over again, we know the result of that—no change, no scary. Maybe staying stuck garners us a ton of attention on social media or with our friends or family. We become that person who always has it rough and needs a break—a script we are reading.

We all have bad days. We all have issues. We all make excuses. But when that becomes the Life we live day in, day out—when excuses and drama become the legacy we seem to be leaving? Then it's time to stop. All the attention and social drama in the world won't fix bad conduct, poor habits, and the lies we are telling others and ourselves. All the habits in the world won't heal or hide the past.

But when we throw ourselves into a state of "I am going to take this Life by the horns and do whatever it takes to take myself to where I want to be"; when we start to act, when we stop making excuses; when we stop blaming (or we at least learn to blame effectively); when we grab the Truth Onion and start peeling that *mofo* like a hungry otter—welcome to the magic—things will change.

It won't be perfect. It won't be easy. It also won't happen overnight or even quickly. But change will happen.

When we zealously search for the Truth, we can clearly see the path in front of us. While it may feel hard and impossible to walk, it's not. We can see the way—because it's all lit up and shining—and no longer dark and gray, hopeless and sad. Now, the forward motion is what we need next.

···· Checkpoint 5 ····································

1. Has your perception of *suffering* changed since Checkpoint 3? If so, write down what suffering means to you.

2. Start your own Truth Onion.
   > What is one thing that you perceive and believe to be a Nonsense problem right now?
   > How far can you peel to get to the Truth of this thing?
   > Does it feel like you have reached the True Truth? If not, what else do you think it would take?

3. What is *your* booze?

#TruthOnion #WhatIsYourBooze #YearOfNoNonsense

Everyone Is Doing
the Best They Can

BEFORE WE TALK ABOUT MOVING FORWARD, WE NEED TO TALK ABOUT the Other People. One of the caveats to the "Other People" is that we are the "Other People" to someone else. So it's a two-way street, and what we expect from others, we likewise should expect from ourselves.

I talked about blame earlier. We can use blame to our advantage—we can blame effectively and with higher intention. But plain ole blame, anger and vitriol, bitterness and hate cannot be in our Year of No Nonsense wheelhouses.

Our duty to ourselves is one thing.

Our duty to the Other People is another.

Depending on our relationship to another person, we have different duties. To our kids, one. To our spouse, another. To our employer, another. To a client or a board, maybe a fiduciary duty.

Duties and obligations are part of Life. Being held captive is not. I would suspect that in about 99.99 percent of all situations in your

Life, you are not being held captive. Maybe you feel like you are in a prison ("marriage is a prison"), but how much of that entrapment is real? How much is manufactured by expectations and lies?

You are, therefore, 99.9 percent capable of walking away, leaving, unfriending, removing, deleting, and saying "no more" to the Other People in your Life. No matter who they are and what relationship you have to them. Will it be easy? Nope. But we do not get to project or blame our own bullshit on the Other People. Simply put, the easiest fix to feeling held captive or that Other People are wronging you is to reframe your own thoughts, expectations, and Core Beliefs.

Sometimes the next fix is to walk away from the relationship entirely. We *do* have that choice. (See Lie 4, Chapter 4.)

Before we dive into the Other People and how to navigate them, it is probably fairly clear that the Year of No Nonsense is mostly about learning to navigate yourself. The Other People are not your problem—unless you allow them to be your problem. Remember the Names we use are important too. (If you call your kids a "problem," then they will most certainly be one.)

I also want to caveat that the Other People may have done some colossal damage that has led us to develop coping mechanisms, addictions, habits, and other destructive things that are "technically" our faults (because we continue to do these destructive things), but also totally a result of the pain or damage from the past. We may just be coming to the place of realizing that we are not broken and we have developed these habits of Nonsense for a *reason*.

The Year of No Nonsense is about recognizing that the Nonsense you are perpetuating came from somewhere—and it may very well be from the Other People who should have loved you and protected you the most. The Nonsense may be from someone who promised to do those things later in Life, and they failed. Nonsense might be business partners and friends; it might be (gasp) family.

Regardless of the Other People—and the destruction they may have left in their wakes—it is now your responsibility to take charge of you. To understand your relationship in orbit with these Other People—to know that you do not rotate around *them*. You do not provide the light of their Universe, and you *cannot*; likewise, they do not provide all *your* light, your existence.

It's a lot, y'all. I get that.

But here's the quick and dirty: most likely, the Nonsense or the perceived issues you have are not with your partner, boss, parents, or kids. I would encourage you to take another look. Some of the Nonsense may have started there, but the *continuation* of it is not because of the Other People. *We* have continued it—on purpose and for a reason—one we may just now be uncovering. We are *seeing* now. Things look different than before.

Therefore, we may need to look again. Stand tall. Accept the Truth.

And take one more look. In *the* mirror. (And maybe another deep breath.)

LOVING PEOPLE

I find loving *all* people a hard thing to do—because I am biased: I have a serious prejudice against assholes. And Other People can be the worst assholes ever—second only to seagulls and ants. But, Houston, we have a problem. *Me* is people too. *You* is people. We are all included in the people pile. Therefore, we are all assholes sometimes.

Other People is a tricky topic for many reasons. After all, the people we love, associate with, and surround ourselves with are a huge part of our lives, our histories, and our futures. That means that even if the people we know aren't necessarily good for us, well, they are still part of us. The Other People have shaped us, instilled their reasoning and politics, Named and Numbered us. So we are somewhat on a mission to untangle ourselves from the Other People—while at the same time, loving them . . . *sheesh*.

I grew up in church, and I know all the right things to say about loving people. But I am also going to be real about it. Someone said to me as a kid, "God knows what you are thinking before you even say it. When you sin, the sin is already in your heart."

Boy, I had a hard time with this one. I mean, when I would get in trouble for speaking my mind or "speaking sin," why was I being punished? If I "sinned" when I *thought* the damn thing, then what the hell was the problem with saying it? God already knew. He (She?) saw the Truth in my little black heart. So what was the big deal?

Well, basically this belief made me a little bit of a jerk as a kid and teenager. Oh, and also as an adult. And maybe still today.

Gossiping and talking shit were next in line to drinking in my list of Nonsense. I think back to "Well if God knows what we are thinking, why not just say it?" And the answer to that is "Because people are *people*. And we should just be kinder." My little sinner heart wasn't the issue as much as hurting Other People.

As a child, I feared God so much that I didn't worry about Other People. We went to a cult church where fire and brimstone was preached ad nauseum and the only book of the Bible taught was Revelation. (Oh, and where we were told that "men are preachers and women can be only be teachers." That one stunk to high heaven for me from a very early age. Perhaps why I love being a speaker, where I'm up on stage just *preaching* away.)

I missed the memo about *Love God, Love People* because it wasn't ever preached. I was just trying not to go to Hell. When you are taught only about Hell, it's probably a struggle to understand the *Love God, Love People* way.

Eventually I learned through trial and error and my own self-teaching and education. *Oh, love is a thing. Got it.*

Fast-forward to that hard year—the Year That Can Kiss My Ass. I had learned to love Other People up until that point, but then I struggled. People hurt me. I decided to just shut down. *Love God, No More People.*

But then I came across a little question. And it single-handedly changed my entire approach to the Other People in my Life, at the grocery, and online.

In her books *Rising Strong* and *Dare to Lead*, Dr. Brené Brown poses this question: "Are people doing the best that they can?"

What is *your* first reaction to this question?

I, like Dr. Brown, immediately thought, "Hell no, people aren't doing the best that they can! People are lazy and slack, and they need to work harder and do better. People suck! People are the worst." *No More People.*

Interestingly though, what we think about the Other People, we often think about ourselves. I struggle immensely with perfectionism. My perfectionistic tendencies drive me into pits of darkness every so often. Because I am not perfect, no one else is being perfect either. When I don't believe I am doing the best I can, I believe Other People aren't either.

Dr. Brown's research reveals, however, that most of us *are* doing the best we personally can. *Whaaaaaat?*

Apparently, because we are mired in our own personal pain and drama, we assume that the Other People are on easy street somehow. We can be reluctant to offer empathy or even kindness. Or perhaps we are able to give grace and compassion to Other People, but we can't stomach giving ourselves the same.

I have a friend, Shelly, who constantly reminds me to give myself Grace. "Give yourself some Grace," she says over and over again. (I actually had to look up the word "Grace" as used in this context and about me and myself.) I finally began to take her advice. Translation: I gave myself a damn break.

For some of us, our best totally sucks from an objective standpoint—but that doesn't mean that it's not our own, personal best.

I put this little experiment into practice for a whole week. Anytime I wanted to lose my shit on someone in traffic, at the store, at home, I just said, "They are doing their best. This is all they have. It's their best. Wow. Their best is truly terrible, but they're giving it. Go them."

(You can't squeeze something out of nothing.)

If someone is doing their best, that's the end of it. I know that sometimes you can't squeeze a bloody ounce more out of me—I am doing my best and then some. Even when I feel like I am not doing my best—if I am lying on the couch watching trash television when I should be working—I say, "Maybe I *need* to be taking a day off. I mean . . . maybe that would make me actually capable of giving my best effort later. Therefore, this is my best."

The problem is that we think our best is some level of perfect. Therefore, we measure our best effort against the best outcome. Those are apples and oranges. We might just be doing our best.

But wait a minute! What about the truly *horrible* people of the world? They're doing the best that they can? *Come on.*

I get it, seems ridiculous. Seems like a lie.

But here's the rub. Asking ourselves "Is everyone doing the best that they can" is more about *us* and how we view the Other People. It simplifies *our* lives; it allows us to focus on *our* Nonsense and not worry about *them*. In other words, if we just assume that everyone is doing the best that they can—then we make our own lives easier. We take the focus off others and place it on what we can control—ourselves, our attitudes. We are no longer rolling in disappointment (because we have expected nothing outside ourselves—an avocado, thanks!). We rely less on the Other People for our own Happiness (and find our own power). People can suck, and their best might just be awful (racist, mean, murderous, and more). So it's a way for us to survive in a world where these (awful) Other People live.

Summary: There may never be a cure-all for the basic asshole or criminal. We can't control them. We can only control the power we give them over us, our thoughts, and how we react to any given situation. Therefore, if we assume everyone is doing their best, we make our own lives easier. We lead better.[1] Live better. We may also give ourselves some Grace. Which is a good thing.

ROMANCE IS DEAD

Lately I see a new romantic pressure to seek (and find) amazing, soul-moving, Life-fulfilling, romantic and sexual love that—like the theory of blissful Happiness—we all deserve.

Soulmates.*

Some idea is swirling that our ultimate needs should be met, catered to, and fulfilled by our soulmate, one special person *made for us* to fill this hole in our soul.

Translation: We are looking for one person to fulfill our deepest needs and inadequacies.

Reality: Who in the world can do that? *Poor bastard. No pressure, Bud or Babe.*

It's no wonder that it feels like relationships are splitting up these days and everyone is cheating on everyone. Of course, that's not true—not everyone is doing anything. But I listened to an interesting TED talk with Esther Perel, who breaks down what infidelity might actually be about.

"Because of this romantic ideal, we are relying on our partner's fidelity with a unique fervor. But we also have never been more inclined to stray, and not because we have new desires today [as opposed to years ago], but [rather] because we live in an era where we feel that we are entitled to pursue our desires, because this is the culture where 'I deserve to be happy.'"[2]

Ah ha, sounds familiar doesn't it.

---

* Like "Good Girl," the term "Soulmate" should never be used. Except in the movie *Good Will Hunting*; that movie is so amazing, they can do whatever they want.

A successful romantic relationship, when you see that mystical, rare creature, consists of two people who stand alone first, as individuals, and then together as a couple. We need to be a stand-alone person, firing on all (or most) cylinders, before we can be anything valuable to anyone else. Many of us have relied on someone else for our validation, existence, and Happiness for much of our Life. If it was our parents' love and attention, that could have been devastating—depending on the appropriate or inappropriate parental roles. If the parents crossed any sort of boundaries in raising you, then likely you get to enjoy a series of issues in romantic relationships. Or, we are looking to heal the dark parental wound, and looking for saving in romantic love. It starts out good, but no one can actually fill that role—not completely.

When someone "fails" us, we then blame them and break up our families for it. And maybe divorce or Splitsville is the complete, 100 percent right call for some relationships. Your Truth Onion might validate that choice fully. No judgments here whatsofreakingever.

But we should not be seeking fulfillment in our own Lives from someone else. Someone else can be the whipped cream and cherry on our banana split sundae. They can be the nuts (or have the nuts). But they cannot be the ice cream. The ice cream is what matters most in the sundae. Without the ice cream, it's just a banana with some whipped cream. *You are the damn ice cream.*

The handful of times my marriage was rocky (translation: damn near almost ended) had almost everything to do with me and very little to do with my husband.

But "He isn't doing x, y, and z!" I was screaming in my head.

No, no he wasn't. He wasn't perfect.

But I had so many issues swirling around, generating a bad attitude and bad actions—how could *anyone* fill the messy, shitty holes that I was making in my own Life? No way. Not even the guy I had dubbed "The Expert."

Coincidentally, this was around the same time that I was doing things that caused the man to leave notes on the counter that said, "You need to get your shit together."

Relationships are beyond complicated and beyond the scope of this book. But I will say that when we work on ourselves, we can see our relationships—and the reasonable or unreasonable pressures we place on them—for what they truly are. Before we look to the Other People as the problem, we might come to understand that where we ourselves are positioned in the relationship might be causing some (even most) of the issues. We might be setting unreasonable expectations of the Other People—and maybe they are doing the best that they can. And maybe so are you.

But seriously, can we ditch the soulmate ideal? Be your own damn soulmate.

THE NONSENSE OF HATE

We live in a world where there is so much hate for different cultures, races, sexual orientations, and gender identifications. I don't know why, except humans tend to dislike people who aren't like them or who challenge their expectations and assumptions (*ah-hem*, Core Beliefs from childhood?).

There is also the age-old adage *People can be assholes*. I'm not sure how old that is—but it's certainly real. And assholes, we all can be. But where I get confused is why would we *not* try to be less of one?

As Malcolm Gladwell points out in *Blink*, maybe we can't help our inherent, deep-seated biases. We have them; they are part of our internal belief systems—right, wrong, or indifferent. However, just because we notice differences in people does not mean we are racists or homophobes; rather, it's the snap judgments that linger longer and influence our behavior and choices surrounding these "thin-sliced" judgments that should bother us.[3]

The judgments and actions that follow are wherein the deep, dark Nonsense of hate and racism lie. The snap judgments are the things that we should (must!) work to overcome and expand beyond. At minimum, to eliminate some of the Nonsense, we need to at least be cognizant of these judgments.

You could have grown up in Albuquerque or New York or San Francisco or Asia. Regardless of our snap biases and history, we can work to change the way we think about Other People. We can look differently at people who are different despite what the past says. That type of change requires deliberate concentration and focus. We are very much influenced by certain Core Beliefs—even insidious, subconscious ones. But in those moments of trying to be different and overcoming, change is occurring.

One of the things I always heard as an excuse for racism growing up was, "You haven't been in the real world, Meredith. There's a *reason* for hating _____." Fill in the blank with the unlike-us-group of the day.*

Love God, Love People.

Hate based on skin color, ethnicity, sexual orientation, religion, or any other thing (really) is Nonsense. I want to emphasize that this is a fundamental form of Nonsense. *Love God, Love People.* (*If you're an atheist, then Love Dogs, Love People.*)

Do we have some of this Nonsense in our lives? Perhaps. Most likely, yes. Is it intentional? Probably not. Maybe. Maybe not.

It's time to fix this Nonsense, even if it's unintentional, because the bigger world is at stake. Our future and our children's and students' biases and beliefs are at stake.

SOCIAL MEDIA LESSONS

Social media is the watering hole of Nonsense.

---

* That is a tough belief to overcome. But it can be done. I, and many of my generation, are proof.

If in doubt about whether or not you should post something on social media—particularly in response to someone else's strong (or idiotic or both) opinion—I have learned this: just don't. I choose to stay quiet and enjoy the rest of my evening. I have never left Twitter feeling refreshed or enriched. Not once—and I love social media. Rather, I leave paranoid, politically tired, and in awe of how no one understands the difference between "your" and "you're."

Why are we even doing social media, we might ask? For me, social media is fun, beautiful, and a way to connect with people we would never know otherwise. I love that part. I love seeing the kittens and babies and sports antics.

Social media's dark side, however, is the cowardice and vitriol that people will spew from their phones and computers but not from their mouths. They'd never say this stuff to your face.

Much like the question about whether everyone is doing the best they can, I have another series of questions that I go back to when it comes to deciding whether to engage, comment, or post on social media.

My current engagement on social media is 100 percent purposeful. I try to put out content or updates, but I rarely post comments or "status updates." I will say positive things ("happy birthday" and "your baby is the cutest thing ever"), but you will not find me fighting people on social media anymore or posting things for mere reactions. I simply won't do it. Of course, there are always a few exceptions. Sometimes the fights are not Nonsense, after all. Sometimes you should fight. But learning to find the line is important.

I no longer post anything when the goal is to try to make someone else look stupid. I have learned my lessons several times over the recent years. I hold my posts, my typing fingers, and my comments to a new standard.

And the greatest gift? It has made *me* so much happier.

If you don't do it for anyone else, do it for your own damn sanity.

I ask these questions now before posting or commenting on social media:

> Is this post helpful to someone?
>
> Am I making someone else feel better with it (or just myself)?
>
> Is it, at a minimum, entertaining in some way?
>
> Even if entertaining, who might this hurt?
>
> Am I being respectful, even if I disagree?
>
> What are the repercussions of this post, comment, or statement?
>
> Is this "share" actually true or from a credible source?
>
> If I post this, will I waste an ungodly amount of time responding to comments about it?

The last one is my guiding light.

Even if I feel something with everything I have, if dealing with my opinion being out there will waste my time, I don't post. Time is valuable, and I am not in the business of wasting mine.

Even if something is true, maybe we don't need to speak it. (Conversely, maybe we do.) If we will lose true friends or loyal followers (who mean something to us), then we should think twice. Now, I don't believe every post should be some massive value-added proposition. Nothing is more annoying than people trying to post something "huge" and "valuable" and "vulnerable" each time. Vulnerable and honest is awesome—but we can go crazy with that also. It's important to remember that social media can be funny, silly, and whimsical as well as valuable. Finding that line, however, is tough—and sometimes we just don't know where we fall. We do, however, learn as we go.

Under some circumstances, we can't ask these questions because the stakes are too high. Maybe someone caused a ruckus about one of our children or our reputation. That's when we find the need to stand up for ourselves—because our reputation, the Truth, or something bigger might be on the line. Many people (especially on the topic of politics) use this "pen is mightier than the sword" tactic in everything they touch online. In reality, your presence on social media should aim to reflect *some sort of mental stability and sanity.* And if we are one of those people constantly flying off the handle, we're only making our own lives especially difficult, and everyone around us likely thinks we are in need of a psych evaluation.

Unless the fire is blazing out of control and your entire Life is being destroyed, take a few minutes and consider the response before you post it. I often write a response in the "notes" app on my phone. I think about it. I ask the questions above.

And if I feel good about it, then I post.

Finally, I learned to turn off my notifications—unless they pertain to a program I am running or something of a more urgent nature. We will be beaten with notifications if we don't turn these off. Choose carefully what hits you. Make sure you are the ruler of your social media time—that you choose when and how you see things.

By asking a few simple questions before our fingers start flying, we can save ourselves a lot of trouble.

But what, you might ask, about the Other People who are causing issues? More on this later.

So what is Nonsense on social media? That's up to you.

But I am certain that spending hours in a given day defending, responding, and reading responses to something you wrote—that perhaps should have been left off social media to begin with—is a giant waste of time. Wasting time is Nonsense. We've got better things to do.

···· **Checkpoint 6** ···

1. Repeat after me: Everyone is doing the best that
    they can. Use this; believe it. Remember it doesn't
    matter if it's actually true or not about a given
    person; this is a way for *you* to Live in the world
    with all these Other People in it.

2. What known biases or prejudices do you have?
    Become aware of them and work to obliterate
    them. In the trying, you are doing.

3. Look at the questions in the box on page 138 be-
    fore you post on social media—adopt them and
    be happier. Are there any that you can add?

#BeYourOwnDamnSoulmate #SocialMediaManners
#NonsenseWateringHole #YearOfNoNonsense
#YouAreTheIceCream

_7_

Cut Out the Bad Wood

_I_ N 2010 SWIM BIKE MOM BEGAN AS A BLOG-JOURNAL OF MY triathlon musings and adventures. I had no idea that it would become a place for people to go to figure out how to do a triathlon and create Life change. That became a big responsibility and one that I was—in no way—prepared for.

For a stretch, I lost my way. I stopped doing it for me, and I tried to make all the Other people like me. Then, when they didn't like me, I got mad and hurt and annoyed. And I considered quitting it all. Well this is a handy recipe for one helluva cake: people pleasing (making all the people like me) + blame (_Why don't all those people like me??_) + failure (_Fine. I quit._).

But I realized that the way the Other People were? That wasn't about me. It was always about them. I was here to Live my Life—to be present in the now—share my story, my feelings, hope it helped someone, and spread my day-to-day hacks. That's it. I wasn't on this planet to babysit or feed drama. I wasn't here to feed excuses, mine or anyone else's. I was here to tell my Truth and perhaps help others to see theirs. I wasn't here to be a pushover either.

I learned a lot of lessons to get there though. Many hard ones. In order to open my heart wide, I needed to also close my circle. In order to close my circle, I needed to open my eyes. In order to open my eyes, I had to come to a place of Truth. And when I did, I could see Nonsense standing out, clear as day.

Once I could *see*, then I began to eliminate the Nonsense—the Other People included. In order for me to continue to Live. To get there, I had to recognize that what everyone thought about me had nothing to do with me.

PEOPLE, PLEASE(ING)

I've spent my Life perfecting the fine art of "people pleasing."

External validation, to this day, is a big part of what keeps my heart beating. Sad, but true. A fine line exists between healthy people pleasing and making yourself absolutely miserable, a model-clay-like replica of some distant version of yourself.

People pleasing is easily defined as putting the needs (actual or emotional—or both) of others above your own—in a habitual or neurotic manner. And it doesn't matter *who* the people are necessarily. That's my definition, not *Psychology Today*'s.

People pleasing has deep roots in our childhoods, which is why I spent so much time talking about childhood earlier. Seeing parts of our past and our relationship to our parents will explain a lot in regard to our current behaviors and people pleasing with the Other People. If growing up, you heard the word "proud" a lot—that should set off some bells of familiarity.

When my kiddos were babies and we would go to a restaurant, you could find me crawling under the table picking up dropped food with my hands before we left. Never mind that I was on *all fours* in a restaurant; I just couldn't leave it messy. *What would the restaurant staff think of me? What would the neighboring diners think?*

The one time I chose to leave the four or five piles of crumbs (and only because I was wearing a skirt), I looked back at the table, and my mom was crouched down, picking up the tortilla chips. *Apple. Tree.* It might seem considerate, but it's insane. Restaurants have brooms and mops; I was using my hands—my near-sixty-year-old mother was then using *hers*. Not that I didn't think about bringing a portable broom and dustpan in my diaper bag. (Totally did.) But why did I not have the "moving on" gene—where I could tip the waitstaff well, leave a "thank you and sorry we're so messy" note, and be just fine? It was not in my DNA.

While I love my husband, I got hitched (at age twenty-one) because I wanted to make everyone happy and proud (and I also wanted freedom, paradoxically—leading to the impossible hurdle of *marriage is a prison*). It never once occurred to me to just Live on my own, make my own money, pay my own rent, do what I damn well pleased, and see what happened. Or to (gasp!) move in with the guy and see how we did as a couple. *That would not have made people proud. Danger, danger.* I made an entire career change because I wanted Other People to think I was successful or important enough to make good money. I got pregnant at the time I did because of the pressure to produce offspring. *Clock was ticking.* By the time I was thirty-one years old, with a career making me anxious, two kids, and a pile of debt, I realized that while the Other People were oh-so-pleased with my choices or didn't give a shit about them, I was turning into a disastrous version of myself.

Now, don't get me wrong. I am not blaming. No one forced me to do anything. *Choices.* But I had Core Beliefs that I acquired, and they influenced me. Making people proud was part of my identity. So my constant focus on proud felt like a strong hand directing me on my *correct* path. Most of my Life I felt a strong hand—parental pressures can be very real and very damaging. Sometimes we don't realize it until way late in Life. Certain things were expected of me from a young age and so engrained that I didn't know how to Live otherwise. So, like a robot, I did the things that fulfilled the needs of others instead of thinking, "Hey. What would I like to do? What would fulfill my needs?"

I carefully use the word "proud" in parenting my kids. I try not to say it at all—or if I do, I remind my kids to make themselves proud, that they are their own barometers of pride. *You did great! Are you proud of yourself?* For a tragically long time, I have needed to make the Other People proud—whoever was looking. By the time I realized that I couldn't often Live up to the imaginary or real expectations, I drank more and more heavily. I grew more and more angry. My anger grew, my belly grew. Everything was growing except the good things, the sense of fulfillment and even a smidge of self-worth.

Unraveling people pleasing is a huge task. Huge. People pleasing may be one of your biggest Nonsense items. I sure as hell know it's one of mine—to this day. My hesitancy to use four-letter words in this book (and in the title!?) was only because of *what will people think?* But the truth is, I Love God, mostly Love People, and say bad words all the time. So getting closer to my Truth usually comes with a side of f-bombs. Perhaps I should temper my tongue a little—sure. But who says? It's mostly the *Other People* who have an issue with it (God loves me anyway). So cussing in public and in this book, while offensive to some of you, is a powerful move for me—it's me moving away from people pleasing in a strong way.

You're fucking welcome.

Staying employed in a job that is killing our soul is an extreme form of people pleasing (or golden handcuffs, *samesies*). We often stay stuck in our jobs because we feel that we must remain there for whatever reason—Fear, money, status, education, and on and on. Working and remaining miserable is, in some way, people pleasing.

We can strive to handle all relationships and people with kindness, respect, and care. We can take a step back from people pleasing and speaking like a sailor but also keep our boundaries. (We can also not be a judgmental jerk about authors who cuss in books.) We have a choice in all these things.

We must ask who we are attempting to please and why. Mostly why. Why does it matter what this person thinks about me? Well, for a boss to like you, that's a big thing—you probably need to keep your job (unless you really don't—as in the circumstance above). But if your people pleasing is out of control, it might actually impact your Health.

Sherry Pagoto, PhD, writes, "A People Pleaser is one of the nicest and most helpful people you know. They never say 'no.' You can always count on them for a favor. In fact, they spend a great deal of time doing things for other people. They get their work done, help others with their work, make all the plans, and are always there for family members and friends. . . . Unfortunately, it can be an extremely unhealthy pattern of behavior."[1]

So why are we exhibiting the people-pleasing behavior? Well, it appears to stem from good old Fear: a Fear of rejection or a Fear of failure. The Fear of rejection shows up as "If I don't do everything I can to make this person happy, they might leave or stop caring for me." This may arise from early relationships where love was "conditional or in which you were rejected/abandoned by an important person in your Life (parent left or was emotionally unavailable or inconsistently available)."[2]

The Fear of failure can be defined as "If I make a mistake, I will disappoint people and/or be punished." Pagoto writes that "people who had highly critical parents may develop a people-pleasing pattern." "Even though the parent or other important person in your Life who doled out the criticism may no longer be in your Life" or the conflict has been addressed and resolved, anxiety surrounding this situation can endure.

Oftentimes "to deal with that anxiety, we do everything we can to get things right, finish the job, and make sure everybody is happy."[3]

Um. Ouch.

Our time in a day is finite—and even though we all have the same twenty-four hours—if we spend all of it appeasing others, then we won't have much time (or energy) to pursue our needs and Dreams. People pleasing may be habitual: we may have spent our Lives yielding to the needs of the Other People. So much that we don't even know the needs we have. Worse, we may not even realize this is happening. The feeling of compliance is just there—that we have emptiness and unmet needs. Like many things, we have no idea where it started (most likely childhood). We just know that we have silently built up sadness, depression, and resentment—despite feeling that we had this golden childhood and should just say "hashtag blessed."[4] This resentment may take years and years to build, but in the aftermath, we have grown addicted or bitter, negative, and passive-aggressive. We might become social media nightmares or Mommy Dearests. Because we are harboring resentment and anger, we struggle to nurture real, productive relationships; we fail as partners, productive employees, and parents. Negativity and aggression, even if kept at bay from the Other People, will surface in the form of distractions, procrastination, or the simple inability to be present and productive.

The people-pleasing monster is fed by the concept of "busy." People pleasers are the busiest people you will ever meet. Because we gain our importance from fulfilling the needs of others, we are too busy to care for our own needs. Likewise, we develop weight problems and destructive behaviors because we've spent all our energy being busy—we "just don't have time for" our own Health.

People pleasers have an especially hard time telling people to piss off.

Highly sensitive people, or *empaths*, can take people pleasing and poor boundary setting to another level. Often characterized as introverts, empaths can be sensitive to sounds, sights, and smells. Highly sensitive people in general need more time alone, especially after a busy day; they need quiet time to recharge. Empaths, however, have been said to share these traits, but they go a step beyond: they can sense and absorb energy from Other People into their own bodies. Empaths then experience emotional energy and physical sensations in very deep ways, such as "energetically internaliz[ing] the feelings and pain of others—and often [having] trouble distinguishing someone else's discomfort" from their own.[5]

Is there such a thing as healthy people pleasing? Sure. It's honorable that we want to make our families, our bosses, our kids, and our country proud. The issue is when we do it at the *expense* of ourselves, at the expense of our own Health, goals, and sanity. Getting to the reasons why we are doing all this people pleasing takes us back to the Truth Onion. We need to ask the right questions and peel.

One of the greatest forms of Nonsense is putting ourselves in situations that continue to feed our sadness, depression, addiction, or neurosis. The "why" behind our neurosis matters big time if we want to get to the heart of it all. But even if we don't want to go trekking into the past, we can recognize that the people-pleasing Nonsense is not helping us be our best selves.

Our light is dimmed so that someone else's can shine brighter.

If this feels like you, then it's time to turn up your bulbs. Or perhaps, your bulbs are plenty bright—you're just shining in the wrong room.

BOUNDARIES: NOT JUST FOR SPORTS

If we have shitty opinions of ourselves coupled with a people-pleasing tendency, we easily allow people to run right over us. *Pushover, beep beep.* The distinction between a people pleaser and a pushover is a fuzzy little line. If you are a people pleaser, you can't stomach being *disliked*. Because being disliked *stings*. So we do things that make the Other People happy in order to be liked, even by people *we* don't like—and we are making ourselves these angry little pushovers. We often know we are doing it; yet we can't seem to let it go. When we are busy making everyone else happy, we are likely saying yes—all the time. Shonda Rimes, in her incredible book *The Year of Yes*, talks about how she forced her introverted self to say yes—yes to parties, events, opportunities, and people—because she had a chronic habit of saying no for so long.

(Shonda was *not* a people pleaser.) Non–people pleasers work to teach themselves to say yes.

People pleasers need to learn to say no.

We may have no established boundaries when it comes to how people treat us or how we allow ourselves to be treated (perhaps a better way to frame it). We deem ourselves not worthy of better; we learn to accept the way others treat us as the norm. Sometimes we don't even realize that we've been treated poorly or destructively or have been victims of emotional abuse—for our whole lives. Then we treat ourselves just as poorly as the Other People have done—if not worse. But when we know that this behavior or abuse has happened, when we see—we suddenly understand that we have a choice to accept this treatment or not. *We get what we tolerate.*

We must learn to set boundaries for what we will accept from others. We must learn to set boundaries for what we will accept from ourselves!!!! (Holy crap, I hate exclamation marks. So let me tell you how purposeful that last statement was. [!])

Once we put up a boundary, we then must stick to it (unless it's a stupid boundary; then reassess). Which is hard. Very, because boundaries will be particularly troublesome when everyone is accustomed to your pleasing them. The Other People might express their "disappointment" (oh, that's the *worst* for a people pleaser!). It doesn't matter. Let them be disappointed in your choices. Deal with it—it's okay. "You're a grown damn adult," someone once said to me. No reason to feel guilty.

Boundaries can include simple things like learning to say no in situations that are hard: cooking for the entire family all the time, volunteering at the school. Or the boundaries can be massive walls to protect ourselves—cutting people out of our lives, removing ourselves from bad situations and limiting our "exposure" to certain people.

I heard the term "Energy Vampire" from Oprah over two decades ago, and immediately a few people popped into my mind. I knew the Energy Vampires in my Life instantly. Toxic relationships run the gamut from snarkiness to tragic forms of abuse to emotional garbage to the ever-annoying "frenemy." With social media, we may have toxic friendships and relationships over the internet. Or rather, we are enduring people that we shouldn't. Fifteen years ago, if you moved to another town and didn't like certain people, you didn't *see* them. Like, ever. Now? Hell no. They show up on your suggested friends page. I keep hoping for the "When Hell Freezes Over" response to friend requests.

How we position ourselves in relation to Other People is where our "Other People" conflicts often arise. What behaviors in Other People do we encourage, enable, and tolerate? What treatment or lies about us and these relationships do we facilitate, accept, and further? What habits and impulses with regard to people do we visit and revisit?

Toxic relationships and friendships did not become a thing for me until much later in Life. Because I didn't realize I had been dealing with people pleasing my entire Life. Read: I had been too busy pleasing the Other People to realize it.

The following is an easy question to ask when dealing with the Other People:

Does spending time with this Other Person make *me* a better person?

In other words, do you gain something from it? Do you feel recharged or inspired? Simply, do you enjoy your time with them? Is the time spent worth it?

I realized that spending time with this one friend, Kathy, a few years back made me a worse person. And maybe that was my insecurity talking. But it was true. (Is it true? Yes or no. Yes, being around Kathy made me sort of homicidal and nuts.) I left Kathy's company feeling panicked and competitive, like I was in a race to nowhere and I better get there quickly. I felt like I was constantly explaining myself. I was tired after leaving. I felt fatter and lazier. Regardless of whether this was my lack of self-esteem or not, I was certain that I did not leave my interactions with her a better person. I left her presence drained and manic.

I realized this question extended to others as well. When I spent time with certain people, I would leave anxious and angry. Spending time with those folks went back to my people-pleasing roots. I was so deep in people pleasing that I wanted to please people I didn't even like. That is some stupid shiznit right there. It seems ludicrous that I had to peel any sort of Truth Onion to get to that crazy core. But I had to work and peel to uncover these Truths. You may need to also.

WE DON'T ASK. AND WE DON'T WORK (THAT) HARD. (BUT WE'RE DOING THE BEST WE CAN.)

Right when I was about to negotiate the salary for my first job as an attorney, I read *Women Don't Ask*.[6] I learned that generally women stink at negotiating because they *don't ask for what they want. Women don't ask. We want to be polite. We believe we aren't worthy of more.*

It may be simpler than this, though. We don't ask, and it goes back to people pleasing. We don't even recognize that we have legitimate *needs*—many of which are unmet—because we have been too busy meeting the needs of the Other People. Therefore, we need to ask ourselves: What do I need? What do I want?*

So, yes, I read the book on asking for what I wanted, and therefore I was ready to negotiate my first salary. However, the demand for lawyers began its slow and steady decline the year I graduated. I was a middle-of-the-class law student, which meant that I had a hard time getting a job (most mid to large firms want the top-of-the-class students). Worse than that, I was overweight and probably smelled like booze in the interviews. I blamed my size for not landing the jobs, and it can be a real barrier, no matter what people say. But also, smelling like vodka and looking hungover—probably a larger barrier.

So when I was offered a job in a small town making less than I would have waiting tables at a fancy restaurant, I asked for more.

And the boss said, "No."

And I said, "Well, alrighty then," and took the job. I wanted more, but also knew that some money was better than no money. I also had the sneaking suspicion that I wasn't worthy of more at this time either. *Inverted. Or something.*

A few years later, I applied for a bigger law job in a bigger city. I had a great interview with the firm, and they offered me a fair salary—and maternity leave (did I mention I was five months pregnant?). But it just wasn't enough for the move, cost of living, and circumstances (new baby). Yes, it was better than the other job. But I wouldn't have felt good about it. And yes, I *did* have a salary in mind that would make it worth the change.

---

*We may not even know our needs. But here's a starting list of needs that might resonate with you: affection, appreciation, community, consistency, intimacy, safety, warmth, authenticity, joy, competence, challenge, freedom, clarity, growth, rest, exercise, and presence. Which of these aren't you receiving despite needing it? Which aren't on the list?

So I asked. Pregnant and desperate, I still had a sense that I needed more. I wanted more. I swung for the fence, and I got the job and the salary I asked for. I had maternity leave, and it was wonderful.

I worked for this hiring attorney for almost nine of the twelve years I practiced law—in different roles and firms—but always with her. I was grateful; I owed her so much. She was a mentor, a friend, and one of the main reasons I stayed in law for as long as I did. (The people I loved; the profession became the stickler for me.)

I learned that even though asking may feel hard, I can do it—simply ask for what I want, need, or desire.

And the Other People? They can simply say no. That is Truth.

When we have a certain idea of what we need to succeed or make our lives work, and we don't get the things we need, then we are setting ourselves up for failure—in some sense. Again, we need to know what we want or need first. I had a hard time believing that I was *worth* certain things. But I reframed my needs as "things I need to make my Life work" instead of my *personal* needs. I wouldn't do that now. I wholly admit that I want the things I want and need the things I need.

But back then, it made the asking easier. Take whatever stance is necessary to ask—just remember to ask.

Cutting out the bad wood in Life is more than just cutting out toxic relationships or setting boundaries with the Other People. Bad wood can also be the Core Beliefs that harm us, the Nonsense we are tending to. Bad wood *is* Nonsense. When we don't ask for what we want or need, that's hauling around some bad wood, with potential for dangerous resentment and bitterness. Cut it. Start asking.

First, if we are disgruntled about not having what we need/want, we become angry and less productive. Employers, friends, or others might not even know we want this thing we want. They aren't mind readers. We can easily find ourselves resenting them, and they have no idea that our internal misery is happening. Next, we can blame—

blame the boss, the family, whoever it seems is suddenly not meeting our needs (mind you, the invisible need we did not discuss—or perhaps cannot even articulate yet). Finally, deciding to ask for *something* is a step toward claiming your worth. If you know you need it, ask for it. If you think you need it, open up a line of communication and talk about it.

Try it. Literally, the worst that can happen is the Other People will say no.

And if that person is an asshole about it? We're moving away from *people pleasing*. Remember? It's their problem, not yours.

I have learned a lot about this by asking "big-name" people to be guests on my podcast. Most of the time they say no, but sometimes they say yes. I happened to email Dr. Shefali Tsabary and asked her to be on the show. She personally emailed me back in five minutes and said, "Can we do it tomorrow?" *Boom. What?* I have asked magazines if I can write for them. Most of the time, I hear nothing. But sometimes they say sure. I ask people if we can have a conversation about something important to them. I have walked up to people and introduced myself. I don't care about asking anyone at this point.

I have learned also that someone is never going to just "give" you something, unless they are philanthropic and it's your lucky day (rare). We must show people what we will give them in return for their commodity—their time or advice or sometimes connections. We must show people the value we bring, the ways we have worked, the sweat and the blood (if necessary).

You must show people what you've got and what you will provide to make their Lives better, easier, funnier. People are generous and kind for the most part, I believe. And we are doing the best that we can. And we'll assume that of Other People. But sometimes you gotta show it. The best, our best, has to be visible.

When I interviewed James Lawrence (aka the "Iron Cowboy") on my show, The Same 24 Hours Podcast,[7] he said something so pertinent to this concept. He is best known for completing fifty iron distance triathlons, in fifty days, in fifty states. He told me, "That's what people know me for. But it took ten years for me to get to the 50-50-50. Most people don't realize how long ten years of work—at one thing—is. How much work it took to get to this one event."

Overnight sensations may exist. But even in the quick rises, we often fail to *see* the years of hard work behind the scenes. Justin Bieber is a great example of a star who seemed to appear out of nowhere. In a documentary, there he was, in diapers, with a guitar. Singing at age three. On stage, performing, at age four. He hit stardom around age thirteen—after he had been hustling with his songs on YouTube. Overnight success? It would seem so. However, that kid had been working for over nine years when he was discovered.[8]

John Grisham, author of best sellers like *The Firm* and *The Client*, spent four years writing his first book, *A Time to Kill*, which was published in 1989. Why did it take him so long? Well, during his writing, he still had his *law* job. The writing was a side hustle, and the rumor is that he wrote a page a day. Upon its completion, the book was rejected by two dozen publishers before Wynwood Press, a relatively unknown publisher, agreed to a 5,000-copy printing. After it was published and even though unsure of the book's success, he immediately began writing *The Firm*. *The Firm* was published in 1991 and stayed on the *New York Times* Best Seller list for over forty weeks, was adapted for film, and launched Grisham to fame. Grisham is one of only a handful of authors in the world to sell 2 million copies on a first printing.

I would have never been ready for any Success at twenty-five. I would have totally blown it—apparently on online gambling and booze. Wisdom, Grace, and stupidity avoidance take time to cultivate. *Emotional Intelligence. Self-Awareness.* And even then, we don't always get it right. Of course, you'll find an exception to every single rule, and yay for the people who work to change the status quo. That being said: experience comes with age, wisdom comes with experience, and keeping our entitled mouths shut until we prove that we know how to work is a big lesson I have learned.

We must learn to cut out the bad wood; to ask for what we want. We also must learn to work—and work hard—for what we want. Finding a balance with our families and the people in our lives is a society-driven goal. But I firmly believe that balance is impossible if we have big enough goals. Something will always be off-balance. So, learning to be off-balance and thriving is the true skill to master. *Balance is bullshit.*

The "big break" is rarely true luck at all—it's the culmination of banging one's head against the wall for a long time, trying to break through—and finally doing so. It's the years and years of hard work, perseverance, and asking questions over and over again. The so-called big break is the *reward* for the hard work.

Not asking for what you want, need, or desire? That's Nonsense.

First make sure you are working. And literally doing the best you can. Then start asking for those things you want. See what happens.

COMPARISON CULTURE

It's not personal. Well, if it involves me, then it's personal. If you hurt my feelings, then it's personal. But what actually isn't personal? Nothing. Everything is personal if it impacts us in some way. (Totally not helpful is it?)

Of the things that we can (and should) control in our Lives, our attitude is pretty much the top thing. We can control the way we allow things to impact us. Sometimes easier said than done. "It's not personal" (as a mantra-type affirmation) only works if it's used for keeping ourselves sane. If that is how we react to someone doing something personally to us. *They are doing the best that they can. It's not personal.* And we move on.

Initially betrayals, lies, pettiness, or cruelty from others may feel fatal, but in Truth? None are fatal. They also may not be personal. The ones wronging us might be doing everything they're doing without a single thought of us. Sometimes that must be true, because it's inconceivable to be on the receiving end of treatment so seemingly unkind.

The meaning and significance that we give these events or actions is what defines their overall and long-standing impact.

So maybe it's not personal. Hmmm. Maybe it depends on what we deem important and how quickly we can right ourselves and move past the wrongs.

Comparing ourselves to the Other People is very personal and tough to handle, especially when we are doing it from a place of inferiority or weakness. For example, we see someone at, perhaps, their best moment on social media, and we compare where we are, perhaps at our current worst moment, wearing crusty pajamas and hungover and alone. There is no point in comparing someone's *years of work* to your beginning or even your middle. The journey—for everyone—is different. The experience is different, the timing, and more.

Deliberate comparison, however, can be a healthy tool.[9] For example, we all have a friend whose Health might be failing in some way. Recognizing gratitude for our Health is a way that deliberate comparison can benefit, ground, and reset us. Additionally, we often come to a place of kindness and helpfulness toward Other People when we look at our Lives through another lens.

One caution, though: our emotions and our feelings, even if they feel a tad crazy sometimes, are *real*, and our suffering is *real*. With deliberate comparison, we can find ourselves in a "someone always has it worse" mentality, leading us to feel that our Hopes, Dreams, and emotions aren't valid or deserving of consideration. People pleasers, especially, must be aware of this habit loop. (See Chapter 5 on suffering).

Comparing ourselves to a former version of ourselves—especially a significantly younger version of ourselves—is toxic as well. For me, this is comparing myself to the former, national-caliber weightlifter Meredith, who could hoist tons of weight over her head. Even comparing myself to the IRONMAN version of Meredith is a trap. Because I was training twenty to thirty hours a week—now, I work out about eight hours. Of course, I will not be in the same shape. *I am a lazy, out-of-shape piece of shit.* (Is it true? Yes or no.)

A constant self-reminder I use is *I am not her. She is also not me.* (Isn't she lucky!?—No! Scratch that.)

When I find myself getting jealous or comparison-y with some other person, I take a step back and remind myself that I can't be her, because I am not her. I have a different Life, body, and soul. I have different talents and issues, strengths and weaknesses. Simply, I am me.

An awesome tool I have uncovered over the last year has been morning journaling. I don't write for long—usually two to three minutes—and I simply go by the format of *The Five-Minute Journal* (www.intelligentchange.com). Loosely, what are three things I am thankful for, three things that would make today great, and two positive affirmations. Then in the evening, I go over what went well and how it could have been better.

Usually the things I am thankful for? Coffee, sleep, and my Health. Simple. But when I first wake up? I am grateful for coffee. The end.

Then I move on to "three things that would make today great": being kind, accomplishing _____ (I write in a daily goal), and being in control of my exercise and nutrition (petty maybe, but it has helped with my binge eating).

Finally, the positive affirmations. These are the big ones. *The Five-Minute Journal* instructs that these should relate to something that we want for the future. For example, when I was trying to get a book deal, my affirmation was "I am a successful published author." I made this daily affirmation every single morning for a year, before I even had one (let alone two) book deals.

In other words, I stepped into my affirmations by basically believing them as Truth.

I am a successful published author. *Is it true? Yes or no.* Hell YES!

For a while, I stopped doing the morning journaling. I noticed a huge difference in my day's tasks and outlook. So I consider the journaling a very exceptional tool.

At night, when I reflect on the day, I find that I usually wish that I had been kinder. *Yikes. Hard to love.* That's a theme that I need to consistently work on, because people are a challenge for me. I grew up as an only child. I work by myself from home. I'm a somewhat disgruntled, crusty writer with a lizard for a pet. I have to work on compassion and kindness sometimes.

We must remember to ask the right questions if we use any type of comparison in our Lives. The best way to deal with the comparison beast is to ground ourselves first thing in the morning with our own gratitude, goals, and affirmations. Then, when we are tempted to go down a rabbit hole of comparisons, we know where we are—or at least where we intend to be, where we will be.

Don't forget: *I am not her. She is not me.*

And remember my "frenemy" Kathy—the one who was competitive and who being around made me a worse person because she set off all sorts of triggers for me? Well, one day, I'd had enough. I just stopped talking to her. I blocked her phone number. I blocked her (and several of her ridiculous cronies) on all my social channels. After a few months, the competitiveness I had with her? Gone. The anger I had toward her? Also gone. Because I don't even think about her anymore. *Gone.*

Choosing what we see and whose voices we hear is a powerful trick to living a Year of No Nonsense.

If we are working with terrible people on a daily basis, it might be time to consider a new role at work or a new job entirely. We can, after all, only deal with this bad wood for so long before we start to rot along with it in some way—either becoming like these Other People or shrinking to fit into their world by dimming ourselves.

We can't expect the Other People to change, especially if the beef is ours. That will never work.

· · · · **Checkpoint 7** ·

1. Are you a people pleaser? (Is it true? Yes or no.) Where do you think the people pleasing comes from?

2. What sense of significance does being "busy" give you?

3. What boundaries do you need to set? What is the first step you can take today to begin to implement these boundaries? Now go take that step.

4. What bad wood can you remove—right now? What will it take to start the process of removing it? Now go take that step.

#CutOutTheBadWood #NoMorePeoplePleasing #DoneDimming #YearOfNoNonsense

You Are in Charge of Your Life

HOPE CAN GET US THROUGH SOME HARD TIMES. DREAMS ARE catalysts to move us forward.

But neither Hopes nor Dreams are official modes of transport.

Originally, this chapter was titled "Hopes and Dreams Are for Losers." I determined that to be a little harsh. But here's the thing: Hopes and Dreams get us nowhere on their own. They have no engines; they are merely a part of the car that takes the journey. Hopes and Dreams are powerful *additions* to a Life of work and action—and living in the now. We want Hopes and Dreams, but they are (again) not the ice cream in the banana split. You are the ice cream. These are the cherries and the nuts.

Hopes and Dreams add a little oomph when the going gets tough.

But they don't make us start and grind and persevere like mad. That is us. That is Grit. That is Hustle. That is hard-ass work. That is movement, action, pain, and yes—you may have guessed it—suffering.

MACGYVER DOESN'T KNOW HOPE

Hope, in some circumstances, becomes the only vehicle for many people—but remember, Hope is not a mode of transport. Conversely, sometimes Hope feels like all we have. I recognize that as well. In rare cases of complete powerlessness, perhaps Hope is the path.

But what about MacGyver? MacGyver didn't Hope; he took action.

He never sat back and said, "I hope someone gets me out of this situation where I need to carry several crates of explosives leaking nitroglycerin across a rocky terrain." (He placed the leaking crates on a surface suspended by wagon springs and sand. To absorb the shock from the terrain. Naturally. I figure, though, there had to be a tampon involved. Those things are handy.)[1]

I Hope I can find a new job.

I Hope he doesn't leave me.

I Hope I lose weight.

I Hope I get into graduate school.

I Hope the cancer doesn't spread.

I Hope I have food to eat.

Notice that a few of these are minor—and a few are major. Hope statements are problematic because we really can't do anything with the things we are simply hoping for. We should only use Hope when we are also busy little bees—planning, exploring, figuring, working, and acting on the situation and our lives.

Gary John Bishop, author of Unf*ck Yourself and Stop Doing That Sh*t, said about Hope, "Imagine you get on a plane. . . . [Y]ou're sitting there, 'This is your pilot. We're gonna be taking off in 6 minutes. I HOPE to get you to LA.' [I would then scream] what do you mean you hope to get me to LA!? Are you taking us, or not?!"[2]

Exactly.

Hope is part of Success—but only part. Hope will not breed Success, relief, or forward progress.

WHY *DREAMS* MATTER

We lose our way, because in the busy of Life, we forgot (and continue to forget) about our Dreams. I don't look at Dreams in the froufrou sense—but rather in the what-the-hell-do-you-want type of way. What do you want to do? Spend your time doing? Where do you want to go? Who do you plan to be? We should never underestimate the power of action, vision, and direction—also known as our Dreams.[3]

It's easy to lose our way though. To choose wrong and live with it—determined that we're just stuck forever. We don't even see it happening.

To figure this out, we must learn which Other People and/or Core Beliefs are harming us, recognize the wrong paths we have chosen, and correct our course—as soon as humanly possible.

Why waste another second reading someone else's script for your Life? We need to broadly identify the things that are making messes of our potential, our paths, our Dreams. Without recognizing the Truth, remember, we are spinning our wheels.

We talked about why childhood—as a theory and a whole—matters in Chapter 2. But now . . . let's think about the positive parts of your younger days.

A simple question: What is something that you loved as a kid? What were you going to "be" when you "grew up"? What connection or relevance do those things have to you now? What connection do these things—that you loved as a kid—have to your Hopes and Dreams?

I think back to my childhood, and my first Dream was to be Annie—as in the Annie from the 1982 movie. I didn't want to be a singer—I wanted to be Annie. I wanted to have red hair, sing, and apparently also be adopted by Oliver Warbucks. Pretty simple.

Annie wore a red sweater. Mister Rogers also wore a red sweater. I loved both of them, and I had a red sweater that—at any moment— could be appropriate for my Life as Annie or Mister Rogers. I learned later that I couldn't sing—I truly can't (not a lie)—but there were things that I could emulate from Annie and Fred Rogers. First, I could get red sweaters until kingdom come. I could move my body. I could make up stories and play puppets. I could make Other People feel sad or loved.

My Dream morphed into what I could do with words. Could I write? Could I draw? Create? Since the very beginning, when I say those things were all part of my Dreams, I believe a more accurate description: those were part of my Life, my plan. *The sun will come out tomorrow.*

As young and older adults, when reality or lies set in, we might change our course. Even with a change, the things we liked when we were five or fifteen probably still matter to us a degree. If we are struggling to find our voice, our reason to Live, or our loves again, the easiest place to look may be our younger years. *What did I love? What did I Dream?*

Likewise, Other People's Dreams are not necessarily mine—your Dreams are not mine, mine are not yours. I want to be a good mom, but I don't honestly care to be Super Mom. I want to be a badass writer, but I don't care much about being a chef. And that is okay. (Repeat after me: That. Is. Okay.)

So many times we forget to Dream our dreams, to have our own plans and thoughts. We forget to develop these plans that are our own—not Super Mom's, or our family's. Or, worse, if we do have Dreams, we bury them under a mustache disguise of excuses.

In order to make Hopes and Dreams something more than just fleeting words, we must discover (or rediscover) our real and burning Dreams and *make the pursuit of these Dreams* a priority.

The common theme I see in women, especially moms of human children, is once the kids come, the Dreams they once had often get dumped in the trash. As if to say, *No more time for these shitty Dreams. When will I be able to do these things, the kids are always needing me! I give up. I'll eat this pizza, drink this wine, and hope my partner doesn't try to touch my disgusting body tonight.*

When did we become *disgusting*? When did our Dreams die?

I swear to God, it can happen overnight, and we have no idea it even occurred until one day we don't recognize the reflection in the mirror or the voice coming out of our mouths.

We know we are hurting on the inside and outside and that we feel lost.

We are here to Live. We have to find our Life. Dreams are the things we will be glad we did at the end of Life.

We may be scared to dream because the Dreams are big or it will take forever to reach them. But guess what? The time is going to pass anyway.[4] Might as well Dream—and make those Dreams a priority.

Digging deep and discovering (or rediscovering) how to Live and what we want is what brings us back to ourselves. When we are marching on toward a Dream, we know ourselves. We find power and more strength than ever. The Dream (and what's coming next) is part of change.

DEAL. FIND. OVERCOME.

How we perceive a situation—whether we are "woe is me" or "I'm gonna crack this code"—makes the difference between Success and failure. If we believe we have everything we need in order to make our own way, then we can accomplish our Dreams on very little.

"An old man . . . wanted to dig over his potato garden, but it was very hard work. His only son, who would have helped him, was in prison.

The old man wrote a letter to his son:

"Dear Son, I am feeling pretty bad because it looks like I won't be able to plant my potato garden this year . . . I'm just getting too old to be digging . . . If you were here, all my troubles would be over. I know you would dig the plot for me, if you weren't in prison.

    Love, Dad"

Shortly, the old man received this telegram:

"For Heaven's sake, Dad, don't dig up the garden!! That's where I buried the GUNS!!"

At 4 a.m. the next morning, a dozen FBI agents and local police officers showed up and dug up the entire garden without finding any guns.

Confused, the old man wrote another note to his son telling him what had happened and asked him what to do next.

His son's reply was: "Go ahead and plant your potatoes, Dad. It's the best I could do for you, from here."[5]

RESOURCEFULNESS:

- the ability to deal skillfully and promptly with new situations and difficulties[6]
- the ability to find quick and clever ways to overcome difficulties[7]

The definition of "resourcefulness" is basically a roadmap to becoming more resourceful—the definition itself tells you how to cultivate resourcefulness: deal skillfully and promptly; find quick and clever ways; overcome difficulties.

Deal. Find. Overcome.

We must cultivate the ability to deal, find, and overcome when it comes to situations, issues, and messed up parts of our childhood (and adulthood). We must deal with difficult things. We must be clever and quick. Resourcefulness is being the best YOU version of MacGyver that you can be.

The good news is that all of those skills are inside of you. You use them on a daily basis in some area or another—at work, in the gym, or driving to the mall. Sometimes we simply haven't been aware enough to transfer those skills to our beliefs, Hopes, and Dreams.

What do you already have at your fingertips? Creativity? Passion? Skills? Great hugs? Hard work? Grit? Gusto? Strong legs and glutes?

Resources cannot be the problem.

And if they are, then it's your job to switch that stinking thinking around. Name yourself Martha McResourceful from Checkpoint 2 and get to work on believing you have all the Resources you need. Focus on what you do have. That's how people who have had hard lives get through—they literally focus on what they *have*, not their have *nots*.

For example, as a new mother it was easy to think, "I don't have time because I am always with these kids, and never mind working! How can I possibly work out?" It can be easy to blame children (bosses, parents, friends, spouses) for our not doing what we want or need to do. However, if we think of the kids (or Other People) as a Resource—things will change. For example, we are now in charge of raising or loving or working with humans. Therefore, to show those humans what is possible, we should be the best versions of ourselves. To be the best versions of ourselves, we need to exercise, eat well, and cultivate a habit of giving a shit about our Health. Kids easily become a Resource for motivation, and changes, not a roadblock to Success.

Maybe it doesn't feel that way. If it doesn't, then that's because you haven't changed your mind to look at it that way.

You are in charge of your Life.

Being in charge does not mean that you are in control of your Life, by the way. But you are in charge of your Life.

Here's the thing: You can choose your priorities. You can choose what you view as Resources. You can create your own method to self-healing and self-helping. You can make your own lists. You can choose so many parts of your day and Life. You may not choose what happens to you, but you can always choose how you react, move forward, take action, or tap into your Resources.

 Maybe the choice is between chicken shit and chicken shit's shit . . . but there is always a choice.

Choice coupled with Resources equals Opportunity, Possibility, and *for the love, Go!*

You have things, Resources, that you can call on. What are your Resources?

HUSTLE AND GRIT

A while back at a conference, I listened as a highly successful mom blogger tried to convince a herd of eager, want-to-be-authors to "ditch the Hustle."

I was stunned. I am a player of the Hustle hard game. Hustle got me to where I was. Hard work is a definitive that I can point to and say, "That works." Now, it wasn't this one time either. On social media, there is a new theme of slowing down, an idea that self-care solves everything and "we should all just breathe." I get that—we can all use a little breath and self-care.

But with that sentiment, there is a dark, deceptive theme of stopping the art of the Hustle.

So this particular individual (telling the audience to ditch the Hustle) was absolutely successful because of, not despite, her years of Hustle.

She was successful because she had a passion, worked hard, and spent hours and hours plugging away at her computer; because she took a massive leap of faith and finance and family and worked harder than she ever had imagined. She absolutely Hustled. *Why was she, of all people, now poo-pooing the idea of Hustle?* I didn't get it.

Does luck happen? Sure. I have seen some of the seemingly laziest people in the world catapult to unfathomable fame and deals. But even annoying YouTubers who are making weird slime or unboxing their Amazon orders? Take a few minutes and watch some, if you haven't. The amount of work, production value and expense, and time those YouTube stars spend on their "craft"? Well, it's a huge investment—energy, lighting, equipment, and makeup. It's also pure and simple Hustle.

Something about this new culture of Hustle-phobia doesn't make sense. Since when is hard work and Grit and Hustle a bad thing?

Let's be real. No one (no one!) can Hustle forever. Rest is a good idea. But Hustle is also a good idea. Periods of Hustle, demanding work, and dedication are a part of Success and change. Why are we being told to sit back and not Hustle? Bullshit. You aren't committing to selling your soul to Hustle . . . but don't be afraid of it. Hustle is the Little Engine of Hopes and Dreams. Hustle says, *I think I can I think I can I think I can.* Hustle will outlast Hope any day.

Are you Gritty? Grit and Hustle are a recipe for *pow*—fireworks!

I listened to the audiobook *Grit: The Power of Passion and Perseverance,* by Angela Duckworth, while I was running a slow half marathon in the Cayman Islands. As I ran-walked that race in the stifling Caribbean heat (poor me, I know), I was thinking, *I am a Gritty mofo. Not many people could stand to go this slow.* Comical, but Grit is a powerful thing. When people say, "I just don't have any motivation," they are actually saying, "I don't have any Grit." Which to me also translates to "I don't have any Discipline" and "I don't care to find any."

Interestingly, though, the research by Duckworth supports the idea that Grit is a thing, an intrinsic characteristic that some peeps have and some peeps don't. Well, you might say, "I'm about as Gritty as pudding." Even if you are Gritty as pudding, is there Hope? *Yep.* Turns out you can also develop Grit.

The basic question raised (and the answer hypothesized) by the book: "Why do naturally talented people frequently fail to reach their potential while other far less gifted individuals go on to achieve amazing things? The secret to outstanding achievement is not talent, but a passionate persistence. In other words, Grit."[8]

We can develop *passionate persistence* in our lives. We can become *passionately persistent* about new things, new Dreams, new ventures.

Are we Gritty by nature in all things? That answer is of course not. Who can possibly be passionately persistent about all things? No one, that's who.

Therefore, the proper choosing of our Hopes and Dreams is of fundamental importance. We must choose wisely. We must choose something that we can be passionately persistent about. Once we choose, I would argue, Grit may come next. Are some people Grittier than others? The answer to that, according to the research, is un-equivocally yes.

Take my children, for example. My daughter (the youngest) is a pile of Grit. She is Gritty in her manic pursuit of things from movies to pizza to running to winning. She's so Gritty, she puts sand to shame. From a very young age, she has had an innate passion for moving—running, gymnastics, yoga, and lifting things. She's had a *passionate persistence* for all things active. We could never pick a single sport because she wanted to do them all.

Stella and I watched the CrossFit Games documentary, *The Redeemed and the Dominant*. She knew that I went to CrossFit and lifted weights. She could have cared less in theory. *Mom does all sorts of weird things,* I have heard her say.

But something in her shifted after watching the likes of the strong, successful, and powerful CrossFit women in the movie. Her eyes were wide at Sara Sigmundsdottir, Katrin Davidsdottir, and Tia-Clair Toomey. Stella saw grace, fluidity, strength, poise, and speed in these young and powerful athletes. She found her role models.

Over the next several months, Stella became *passionately persistent* in the pursuit of CrossFit. She may hate CrossFit by the time this book hits the shelves. But the point is, she approaches whatever she believes in with passionate persistence. The Grit is there. It moves and shifts maybe. She just chooses where to place it.

My son seemed different when it came to Grit. I did not (at first) think him Gritty by nature, like Stella. But I learned later that not only was he an example of the cultivation of Grit—but coupled with his Dream, he had the magic of innate Grit—he just needed to discover a Dream or two.

We introduced James to baseball as a five-year-old. He hated it. We made him play because, well, our family philosophy was that the kids were required to play a sport or be active. Any sport, for the love. They could choose, but they must pick one for the time being.

James's choice: "I choose no sport."

So we chose for him. And *aw hell*, did that kid make us pay for it.

Even as a five-year-old, he made his desires known. He would walk up to the plate and swing three times in a row at whatever came at him (even if it was in the dirt or twenty feet overhead) with absolutely no intention of making contact with the ball. Then he would walk back to the dugout, dragging his bat hard in the dirt and glaring at me. Me! Not his dad. Me. The other parents chuckled because, well, it was hilarious. *Funny not funny. Absolutely zero Fs to give about baseball.*

This behavior went on for three seasons. I had *passionate persistence* in my pursuit of *parenting* this kid to play a sport. We decided that we would just tolerate it as parents because, while we didn't expect an MLB star, we did expect sportsmanship, kindness, and some sort of damn effort. He was killing me softly, I'll be honest.

However, something turned in his eight-year-old season. He was hitting the ball. He had friends. He was fielding. He was doing some pitching. *This is amazing*, I thought.

So fast-forward, and a ten-year-old James pitched his first season as a not-so-sure-he-wanted-to-be-a-pitcher pitcher in fall baseball. Irrespective of how he felt about pitching, his debut game on the mound was *extraordinary*. He displayed a maturity in the game beyond anything I had ever imagined, certainly beyond that bat-dragging-little-poophead from the previous season.

The last game of the season—a tournament—our team's "star" pitcher managed to relinquish the lead and load up the bases with no outs. James was called in to pitch. My heart sank, only because he didn't realize that with bases loaded and no outs, he was walking into a shitstorm—because he had been goofing off in the dugout. It was probably for the best that he just walked into it.

He threw solid pitches. The problem with pitches in the strike zone, however, is that they are *excellent* for batters to hit. One after another, the opposing team cracked the bat, run after run scored.

Objectively, I saw this whole scenario was not James's "fault." He was pitching a good game. But because they were losing, he felt he was failing. The coach, rightly, kept him in the game. The character build was in full effect—which is a terrible thing to watch as a parent.

The team rallied a bit, but it was not enough to win. He was visibly devastated.

I read an article long ago about how, after a sporting event with your children, you are not supposed to say a word. And if you do, all you say is "I love watching you play."[9] I have long heeded this advice, especially after the sporting childhood I had—filled with immediate postevent advice, tips, and "should haves." In other words, if the kid wants to talk about the game, he or she will. If it's a rough game, they need time to process. You just tell them that you love to watch them play—period.

After this particular game, neither I nor my husband said any-thing (and we told Stella, "Be quiet! Say nothing to your brother—or else!"). He was quiet on the drive home. He was still visibly upset. But about fifteen minutes passed, and his sister said, "James, I loved watching you play."

Why are my eyes leaking?!? I thought. A few minutes after that James said, "I would like to practice tomorrow."

We were stunned. And all we said was, "Sure." And then I said, "I loved watching you play too, bud."

The following year, we had moved to a new state, and as I "feared," James asked if he could stop playing baseball. With a semi-heavy heart (me, being such a baseball nut), I was actually okay with it. Relieved even, because I knew it wasn't his passion. He had given it a good effort, and it had been many seasons. And as we honored his request, I looked back on the last season and saw him leave baseball with heart, courage, and sportsmanship, just as we'd hoped—there was no more bat dragging.

With those seasons, James proved (importantly—to himself) that he was Gritty—as much as his sister, as much as anyone. He *was* full of Grit. What I also learned is that baseball was clearly not his Dream. And like childhood, the Dreams we have (or don't have) matter.

James is now over one year into digital animation. I had thought he needed to cultivate Grit—I turned out to be super wrong. Because he had Grit. He just didn't have the Gritty Dream zeroed in. Or he was clearly living in the wrong Dream—because of me. I had projected my love of baseball—my fundamental "requirement" that an Atwood kid play a sport—onto him. That was not conscious parenting; that was me using my son to fulfill a need of mine. I recognize that now, and I am regretful for it.

But since leaving baseball, James has created art goals for himself. He has doodled and sketched since he could hold a pen. Now he sits at his computer on his fancy drawing tablet for hours—creating art and characters and learning software programs that I have no idea how to use. He's teaching himself, and he's thriving. He's pursuing his own Happiness, not mine. His Dream. His Grit.

As with many things in Life, I was wrong about him: he is innately Gritty. (He drew the cute onion for this book, BTW.)

Which made me realize that Grit is related very closely to Dreams, to living Life on your terms. Yes, Grit is somewhat innate, and yes, Grit is also gainable.

Grit is *passionate persistence* in pursuit of a goal. Sure, it can be learned. But when we cultivate Grit based on our Dreams—or based on a place of love and Life—then we present ourselves with the magic opportunity to truly thrive. We just need to find (or remember) the Dream—that version of Life—that sets us on fire in order to compound the effect.

We are all Gritty when we are chasing the right Dream.

We are all Gritty when we are living our best Life.

· · · · Checkpoint 8 ·

1. What is your Dream? Yes, really. What do you want in Life? What did you like to do as a kid? If you could do anything with your Life—right now—what would it be?

2. What are two (or ten) Resources you have at
   your disposal? As with Checkpoint I, you *do* have
   Resources. (PS: Again, even if all you can conjure
   is breath and this book, you have them. This book
   even has a section labeled "Resources" at the end.
   So there.) Extra credit: list every Resource you
   can think of.

3. How can you use these Resources to put you on
   the path toward your best Life?

4. Are you Gritty? (The answer is YES!) And if you
   don't consider yourself Gritty, then how can you
   become *passionately persistent* about this Dream?

#PassionatePersistence #GrittyAndAllThat
#GritGraceAndGratitude #YearOfNoNonsense

PART III

GO AFTER THE LIFE YOU WANT

9

Defining Your Health, Happiness, and Success

WE ARE CONSTANTLY DEVELOPING, MANAGING, AND MAINTAINING our own personal brand, whether we know it or not. The brand consists of our reputation, ideals, and the persona that we outwardly project. The problem with seeking out and working toward creating a personal brand is that it's fundamentally based on how others are perceiving you: *Who likes me? Who is sharing my thoughts? Who agrees with me? Who likes my hair?*

When we are seeking to create an image, a brand of ourselves for *the benefit or "likes" of Other People, then we are building a personal brand of Nonsense.* (And this has been going on since long before social media, people. I mean, did you read *The Great Gatsby?*)

When we stop trying to keep up the people pleasing, when we embrace the Hustle and pursue our Dreams, we don't need a brand. Because we have our lives to Live. But when we try to create a person whom we "show" the world, it's easy to lose who we truly are.

All of this is to say that you, most likely, have inadvertently created your own version of a personal brand, whether you are a stay-at-home mom, doctor, engineer, or whatever—and it may (may!) just be a Brand of Nonsense.

 A Brand of Nonsense is that special state of self-imposed equilibrium, no matter how strange, destructive, or impossible, that we believe we must maintain and show for the crowd.

The crowd may be small.

The crowd may be big.

The crowd might be just the people closest to us—from whom we are hiding our struggles, our pain because we don't want to hurt them. The persona we are working on? That's the brand we are creating.

Now, sometimes the brand we work on is fantastic, and it has nothing to do with a crowd.

"I want to be healthy, strong, and working hard toward the career that makes me shine." "I want to be the best mom possible and show my kids what it means to be _____."

Super, dude. There is nothing wrong with changing and morphing into exactly who we want to be. I said we *may* be creating a Brand of Nonsense; doesn't mean we all are.

But unless we are creating a Life that rumbles more like a revolution, a calling, a change, or a reason to Live—then we're just out there making noise. Noise is fun to watch, mind you. I love a good episode of the Kardashians as much as the next person—total noise—but I don't leave any episode as a better person. You might get filthy rich off noise and win at noisemaking. But we certainly don't get rich *watching* it.

We are better than just noise. We can win at Living. And wear our Kardashian-nude lipstick too. High five.

In what's next, you'll learn what your personal Brand of Nonsense looks like. If you are grounded in what you know for sure

(Oprah), then you are more easily able to know what is not part of peeling the Truth Onion (me). You can point and scream, "LIE!" and "NONSENSE!" like an absolute freak, but at least these are the things you know for sure.

IS YOUR LIFE A YARD SALE?

Eight years after my first triathlon blog post on *Swim Bike Mom*, my "personal brand" had exploded out of control. And not in a good way. This was the Year That Can Kiss My Ass—and my Life was a Yard Sale. I had a little bit of everything going on—and sometimes at close-out prices.

I was working to service my audience, but I was trying to service every last person with something that they might need. I was trying to make everyone like me (people pleasing), trying to make everyone happy (childhood). In reality, I simply needed to remember to Live.

With *Swim Bike Mom*, I just wanted to tell women that another path different from sad, unhealthy, mad, depressed, and Dream-less existed. Maybe it was via triathlon, maybe it was something else—but we could all do better than that constant state of sad, worried, and stuck.

I thought back to my childhood Dreams. Did any of those early Dreams look like what I was doing—with my Yard Sale? Not really. But I was close—I was writing, after all. I could feel, hear, and smell it.

I had my toes in the sea of things I wanted—but I was not committing to diving in. I still was hung up on several things. I had not planned well enough financially to leap from the *Swim Bike Mom* "side Hustle" to making a living doing what I loved. I didn't have a real plan either.

Do you have some sort of Yard Sale going on in your Life? Are you expending time and energy in the direction of a million different things and people at close-out prices? Are you watching ideas and Dreams march out of your Life for way less than you paid for them?

In hindsight (of course), one of the best things that could have happened to me was the terrible year, the birthplace of the Year of No Nonsense. In that year, I lost friends, businesses, and reputation. Some of this was my fault, but most of it stemmed from lies and perception out of my control. I received text after text, drama after drama in my inbox. I stayed mostly silent.

But I was reeling.

All the Yard Sale things I had worked so hard for, things I had earned? Much of it seemed to disintegrate in a span of weeks. Then I stood by and watched as it continued to landslide for nearly another year.

And I simply let it go, let it slide. I held onto everything with a loose grip. Things that remained, remained. Things that slid away? Well, they were gone.

After the panic subsided, I looked around at the weird but glorious rubble and thought, "Well, this is interesting." (Then I threw a massive temper tantrum.)

Sometimes we have to look at the situation and be honest (what lies are being told here), then let the Truth anchor us with its giant boulders . . . and allow the sand, soot, and trash to slide through our fingers.

As expected, when Life is challenging, we often head straight for the path of least resistance. But we do that while holding on, death-grip style, to what is left. A conundrum.

The most painful thought during the year of destruction was this: *Had I not gone on a wild goose chase of triathlon. Had I not tried to make a difference in this weird-ass sport. Had I just kept my mouth shut, stayed closed off, I would have been a partner in a random law firm somewhere—like years ago.*

All the time I had spent writing random blog posts that no one read, I could have been printing money as a partner in a firm. I'd be respected instead of a human litterbox. I'd have a Career instead of a Yard Sale. I would have financial stability instead of a clothing business that had bankrupted itself. I would have all my (real) suits and heels instead of leggings and sneakers.

Shoulda. Coulda. Woulda.

But that was a lie too. My Life was never meant to be in the law. I would be building a Brand of Nonsense if I tried.

I was never meant to be Notorious RBG[*]; I was Notorious SBM. I was me. All that regret talk was Nonsense. It was based in Fear. I was holding on to the past of the law while trying to let the rest go. Push, pull, death grip. Fear. I began to see Nonsense (uncertainty, Fear, sadness, betrayal, drama) more clearly for what it was. I knew that I must close up the Yard Sale and have someone chain me to my home office to keep me away from law job interviews. I was having a crisis, and it was all connected to discovering, naming, seeing, and determining to get rid of Nonsense. And it was a glorious, amazing breakdown. Something magical was happening.

The glory was in the breakdown. The sky is the biggest and bluest from rock-freaking-bottom. You may have to break down too, before you can build up.

HHS (HEALTH, HAPPINESS, AND SUCCESS)

Now is time for the hardest part ever: the Self-Inventory.

(Is this true? Yes or no.) Yes. I am sorry, but it's true. We need to get down to the nitty-gritty True Truth Onion about ourselves, our habits, our lives—and that means our Nonsense. Time to dissect the little thing(s) in order to tackle the big thing(s).

Sometimes when things are not going well for us, the world is not to blame. The cause is instead that which is currently most valued, subjectively and personally.[1]

---

[*] Ruth Bader Ginsburg: civil rights attorney; justice of the US Supreme Court, appointed by President Bill Clinton, who took the oath of office on August 10, 1993.

But first, a review of what we have learned until now.

You are on a quest to get rid of Nonsense.

(You *have* Nonsense. You *are not* Nonsense.)

You have been lied to. You lie to yourself.

Childhood matters.

You must *see* the Truth. No matter how ugly the Truth may be.

You may need to *peel* layer after layer to get to the Truth.

Even then, you may need to peel more.

Good and not-so-good things and Other People from your past
   might be driving your current versions of Truth, Core Beliefs,
   habits, and behaviors.

You can Name (or rename) yourself, choose what Numbers define you.

Dreams matter—work on reengaging or chasing yours.

Everyone is doing the best that they can.

Get away from People Pleasing.

You have a Choice.

Hustle is good.

You have Grit.

The Other People are not your problem; boundaries may be.

You have Resources. Therefore, you are Resourceful.

You can block people on social media.

Second, I want to give you a lens to think about what is coming.
The next section is about cracking open *your* Year of No Nonsense,
but before we can begin to change, we need to *see*. To come to know
the Truth.

Maybe you have done that already in earlier chapters, but this is
the new and next rung.

Let's look at ourselves and our Life with a few principles in mind: our
Core Beliefs on the subjects of Health, Happiness, and Success (HHS).

Health

Health is objective. You can have great bloodwork, blood pressure, and a low resting heart rate. You can run a sub-six-minute mile and bench-press your body weight. You can sleep eight hours a day and meditate. Etc.

So, what if you like cage fighting, base jumping, and shark fishing and subsist only on Hungry Man microwave meals? Is that healthy? I don't know. Objectively, I would say probably no.

But who am I to say? Health is also subjective.

What matters to you about your Health—is what matters. For a moment, turn off your awareness of Health Numbers and Names and measurements, body ideals and role models, teammates, coaches, and friends on social media. For a moment, take a second and consider what Health actually means to you.

If you were dropped onto planet Earth today and you didn't speak any language or understand the crazy thing called social media, what would Health feel like? What would you do, as a stranger to Earth, to feel your best? Would you walk a lot, spend time in the sun (with sunscreen, of course)? What would make you feel free, loved, and grounded? As you might suspect, Health is the starting point for Life—but we have forgotten this small fact. Often we think of Health as aesthetics—how we look—or a series of Names and conditions, Numbers and facts.

Health is about how we feel—as a whole person.

If we don't feel well (physically, emotionally, financially, spiritually), we cannot pursue Happiness. (Yes, Happiness is a lie we've been told. More coming. Stay the course.)

If we are too tired, hungover, emotionally in the ditch—we are in a state of paralysis—we perceive ourselves as stuck. Of course, we don't look for a new job or pursue our education or put ourselves out on the dating market—we feel like crap. How could we expect someone to love or hire us—when we aren't even in our own corner? If we don't feel well, any type of Success is meaningless. Also, the desired type of Success will probably not happen.

Unfortunately, we come to the idea of Health with the same biases we have for most everything else. We have stigmas about tattoos, mental Health, nose rings, and torn jeans. We have opinions and shame associated with addiction, suicide attempts, infidelity, and job choice. Pick a "shameful" behavior, and we each have a bias about it. Pick a type of food, and there may be shame behind it. The Number on the scale, skin conditions, the way we look. Our internal biases matter. Leaving our experiences and our biases behind is probably an impossible task. Reprogramming ourselves and our thoughts and working to rid ourselves of our biases takes a virtually insurmountable pile of work—a pile of work that most of us would rather not tackle. But we need to be aware of it—because it ties in to our Health.

Our reactions to social media, politics, and anger at the Other People, road rage and impatience in the checkout line, a fundamental belief that *no one is doing the best that they can*—all this, too, impacts our Health.

Our internal dialogue and thought processes about ourselves and the Other People are very much about our Health. Whether we have dialogue about a kid walking down the street or someone at work or an internal dialogue about ourselves, we are making a mark on our Health.

Unfortunately, and still to this day, my day can be made or broken by the Number on the scale, as I have more or less admitted in the section on "why Numbers hurt." Not gaining weight is a big part of my Health goal that comes from years of programming, weight-based performance sports, and self-loathing.

But the True Truth goes deeper.

My weight is about my worth, and I was measured by it during childhood. It was about love and approval. Food was felt to be about comfort and nurturing; food was then often denied. My weight is deeper than the scale. Yours may be too. That's why "Just Love Yourself!" doesn't work.

The scale, while it cannot be the final barometer of my self-worth and Health, *is* a measure that matters to me. The scale matters to my Health. I must be honest with myself. And being honest is hard. Being honest hurts, disappoints people. I am no longer ashamed.

The scale is a measure that points to the primal wound of my childhood. So I am positioning myself constantly around that bleeding, gaping pain—trying to re-Name, re-Number, and resurrect my true self. The scale is a mere symbol of the things I must overcome—emotionally and spiritually.

The beautiful thing is that I have arrived at my True Truth, and I now know what to do with it. I put the Truth in a place where Truths can go. I have since added *other* measures, other Names, other Numbers to guide my Life with regard to my Health—but I don't ignore the Truth about what Health means to *me*.

So when someone says, "Meredith! Get over the scale. Love yourself."

I can say, with Truth: you literally have no idea what you're talking about. *Eyes on your own plate, Karen.*

And you—no matter what your Truth is—can say the same about your Life. The Other People? What they think is none of our biz.

Truth is an onion—it's complicated and crusty. Truth might be a patch of onions.

To move forward, we must strip away all delusions about Health—as it relates to us. We must come to the table with a fair-minded and nonbiased judgment of our own personal Health, of what Health means and what matters to us. We must not apologize for wanting to change, for wanting more, for having a different version of *Health* than someone else. We have messes made from the past; we have messes inside us (we are not messes)—and we need to figure out those things up front in order to move forward. Not in order to shame ourselves but rather to have an accurate understanding of where our judgments, goals, and desires come from. To help guide us toward what we want.

What do you desire about your Health? What makes you feel like the best version of yourself?

Do you think you are stupid because a teacher told you so?

Do you want to be "skinny" because you had a parent who fat-shamed you?

Do you exercise only to burn off what you ate?

Is your alcohol and/or drug use "no big deal"?

Do you require coffee to wake up and drugs to sleep?

What is Health to you? If you could go "poof"—what would you change?

Happiness (the Pursuit of)

Ask yourself, *What makes me happy?*

Is this a difficult question to answer?

I force myself to answer this question often. When I think of the things that make me truly happy, I have a very short list. Because to me "Happiness" means "bliss." How much of our lives and day do we spend in "bliss"? What gives me blissful moments? Maybe the turn of magical fall weather. When both my kids are bathed, smelling like desserts and snuggling quietly while reading books. A massive personal record on the race course or in the weight room. Those events evoke Happiness in me.

But one thing that they all have in common? Those moments are rare.

That's because bliss—what we really mean with the Happiness idea—is also rare. Contentment, peace, and calm? That is another story—that is truly what we are seeking (see Chapter 3). Those can be daily. They can even be "most of the time"—if we are truly Living.

Next question: *When am I content? When do I feel peaceful?*

My list expands: Sitting with a fresh coffee and cracking open my laptop to work. Working toward the next big idea (pursuit of Happiness). Closing my eyes at night and knowing that I truly gave the day everything I could. Laughing with the kids. Sharing an old joke with my husband. Talking about the glory days of weightlifting with former teammates. Saving $5 at the store. A good workout. A nice, healthy meal. (Also, a solid, gooey grilled cheese.) A book that changes my perspective. Stretching before bed—knowing that I took care of my body before I closed my eyes. Remembering to take the wet clothes out of the washer and put them in the dryer before they smell (win!). Also, knowing I fed myself well, exercised, and stuck to my Health goals for the day. Health is a big part of my contentment, my pursuit of Happiness.

Contentment is a huge playing field. Contentment is reachable with a change in attitude, a focus on gratitude, a change in our state of mind. We can thrive while we are pursuing that rare, magical Happiness bliss by enjoying the proximity of contentment. We can be content and work hard, pursuing that bliss. We need not be complacent to be content.

One of the lies we have been told is that we deserve to be happy all the time (Chapter 3), and that contentment is mediocre. While we are all worthy of love and puppies and rainbows, who actually gets all of that all the time? Who gets PRs in the weight room all the time? Nobody, that's who. But contentment and peace? We can have that, right?

From a starting point, we deserve exactly what? What do we believe we deserve?

We deserve Happiness, sure. But we also will *never have Happiness all the time.* When we make a broad declaration like, "I deserve to be happy!" we are setting a very, very high bar of expectation. Perhaps we deserve way more than we have, but setting the Happiness bar too high is setting ourselves up for an interesting form of failure. That failure (I am not "happy") then leads us to search frantically for Happiness—the end game—instead of learning to grow and enjoy the journey of *pursuing* happiness. Adjusting the expectation of Happiness to the "pursuit of Happiness" changes everything.

Deep down, many of us struggle with the self-inflicted pain of telling ourselves "I do not deserve love and Happiness" or conversely "I want to be happy!" But these are all loosely worded piles of crap that make huge channels of problems in our Lives. We bestow upon ourselves some of the most preventable problems in the world with our sloppy wants and Hopes for "Happiness."

Can we live in a pure state of Happiness? I don't think so. I sure as hell don't, but hey—if you do—you should write a book.

But I believe we can get to contentment, gratitude, peace—for a lot of our waking hours.

Ultimately that state is up to us. Peace, gratitude, contentment are all *practices* that must be cultivated. Hoping for these things is not action. We gotta work toward peace and contentment. And stop defining Happiness in ways that are impossible, unreachable, and tail-chasingly maddening.

Success

Health is subjective. Happiness is subjective. Success is also subjective.

Your definition of Health, Happiness, and Success is completely *yours*.

Okay, so Success.

How many wildly "successful" people in the world have ended their lives? More than we should be able to count. How many successful people have lost everything? Or, by choice, sold everything to travel the world, become a monk, create an entirely new path? Relinquished a "high-powered" gig or profession in pursuit of another walk of Life entirely? Sure, I had a hard time leaving the law.

But once I decided, I was okay with it. But I had several family members with *way* more heartburn about my giving up my "successful image" to pursue the Health and Happiness I so (desperately) needed.

People will forever project their version of Success onto us—that is not our problem. But what we *tolerate* from the Other People becomes our problem.

We must create our own vision of what Success means.

Here's the thing. Success is directly tied to Health and the (pursuit of) Happiness. Without Health and Happiness, we are not a Success—at least not a version of Success that matters. We can have all the world's Success boxes checked—but none of that matters if our personal Health and (pursuit of) Happiness boxes are empty. Empty Health and pursuit of Happiness boxes are exactly why we see amazingly talented, wealthy, and famous people end their lives tragically—Success matters nothing without the other two elements.

I am fairly sure that everyone's initial knee-jerk thought about the term "Success" is that it's fundamentally tied to wealth, fame, and accomplishments. I mean, look at the magazine covers of the "Success" publications—even one by the name *Success*. The covers are graced by individuals who, if not wildly wealthy, are incredible innovators, entrepreneurs, leaders, and the like. Very rarely do you see a solo humanitarian or some kid from down the street who saved someone from drowning.

That doesn't mean we should avoid any version of Success. We should not avoid the idea that we want a piece of it, that we deserve it, or that we can make it happen. (What is your Dream? See Chapter 8.)

The key is making Success, as a concept, work for you. And to do that, we have to strip away the Nonsense of Success. Then we must define what "Success" is for *you*.

I was a "successful" attorney with the 2.5 kids (we have a lizard) and a "big" house in the suburbs. I had a sensible SUV. I had a pedicure and a Louis Vuitton bag. I had arrived. I had reached "the Dream."

But that wasn't my true Dream, and I could not have been more miserable, drunk, or scared.

The Success I was seeking was not my definition of Success. It was Success as I had been led to understand it. Success as put upon me by culture, family, and mores. I thought it was Success because I was healing certain Fears in my family, in my own misled expectations. But my Health was bad. I was not pursuing my Life—there was no joy in the Pursuit of any Life. I was simply trying to make everyone else proud.

Does Success alleviate suffering? Yes. I think it does.

But only if it is your version of Success; the one that feeds (or is fed by) your Health and (pursuit of) Happiness.

HHS are the three areas of our Lives that must be all working together toward a common goal—a Life of Purpose. These goals need not be in sync, or perfect, or all encompassing. Synchronicity needs to happen eventually, but it doesn't always happen at once. We make it happen quicker, though, by having an understanding of our versions of HHS—coupled with a promise to ourselves to get rid of the Nonsense in our Lives.

THE ONE NONSENSE THING

Here we go. Crack your knuckles. Chug some water. Here's how we begin to apply the Year of No Nonsense to your Life.

At this point, you are up to speed on all the Year of No Nonsense things. Maybe you have found some sisterhood or brotherhood in my story. But, regardless, I know that you have identified some Nonsense, even if you don't like a word I've said. Now you have explored what Health and Happiness and Success mean to you.

I implore you to trust your first reactions, your gut for this next part. If you come up with an answer, ask yourself further, *Is this really the answer? What does my gut say? Is it true? Yes or (really yes) or no.*

Now, I want you to spend ten seconds on a very simple question. Yep, ten seconds, maybe less.

I want your knee-jerk reaction.

I want your gut reaction.

Here is the question.

Let's get to the answer.

 What is the biggest Nonsense RIGHT NOW standing in the way of my Health, Happiness, and Success?

What did you see flash before you? Right here, right now. What is it? Don't think.

What is the thing that you do *not* want to deal with?

What is harming your HHS progress, right now?

What is it?

If you have spent some time working through the lies and peeling the Truth Onion(s), then you might arrive at the root of THE thing standing in the way.

If you are in a spiral of negativity, lies, and blame, you may have avoided the real answer to that question like the plague, even subconsciously. You may be far off. You may be on the crusty outer layer of the Truth Onion, or even that slippery next layer, and think you're at the core. You may be through one Truth Onion and need to pick up the next one—like me. (You may be on the potatoes in the next bin over and not even looking at the onions.)

And that's okay, but we need to get to the True Truth core—however hard it is or long that takes. Once you are done with that one, you may need to keep going.

When I first asked myself what "my real issue" was (that was the question at the time), I came up with the following answer. This is what I wrote as the biggest barrier to my Health, Happiness, and Success: *My bodyweight.*

That was it. My weight. (Back to that tired argument, eh? Yes, but wait . . .)

I knew that was BS. I knew, deep down, that my weight had probably 10 percent responsibility for the sadness, depression, feeling of sickness, and regret that I was experiencing on a daily basis. It was present but was not the *cause.* I was intuiting the lies that I had been told for years. I was scratching the surface of the lies I had been telling myself. I saw I was repeating some story, blaming Other People, and there was something about this Truth Onion.

My weight was the top, crusty layer of my Truth Onion.

I knew better. Something other than my weight was the current One Nonsense Thing.

The One Nonsense Thing—*that,* my friends, is what we are after. This is the crux of our current suffering. *Current* suffering. (Meaning that there may always be some, yes.) This is the Thing we must address— no matter how hard, stinky, or unfair—right now—to continue to move toward our greatest HHS, our Dreams.

Was I deeply suffering because I needed to lose twenty or thirty pounds? Of course not. My excess weight itself was not hindering my Life in any way, really. I was slower as a triathlete because of it, but how silly does it seem to list weight as the biggest roadblock to my Health, (pursuit of) Happiness, and Success when I could still run and finish IRONMAN races, sometimes quite well?

But "losing weight" was exactly what I knee-jerked as my biggest issue. Maybe because it was my oldest issue. *Damn inverted childhood.*

If you will notice, being "overweight" isn't on the giant scroll of types of Nonsense I provided. Because the act of being overweight itself isn't really Nonsense; rather it's arguably an impact of behavior and habit on your personal HHS. If being overweight impacts you *not,* then it's not an issue for you. Then it falls under none of the Other People's business. *Eyes on your own plate.*

So what is your One Nonsense Thing, when you ask this question? Dig a little more. What is the action, habit, or thing that is the *cause* of what you are declaring Nonsense? Because that is the real Nonsense.

We focus on the Trees (being overweight, or broke, or lonely) because we don't want to see the Forest (what got us there—maybe something as dark as trauma or abuse—what is keeping us there, what need or identity or story all of these things serve in our Lives).

The Forest (the Truth) scares us. The Forest (which contains the clues to claw our way out of our suffering) has implications about our past, present, and future. The Forest shows us the way and reveals what we must do—so we don't want to focus on that. We'd rather see the Trees. The Trees keep us very busy, with all their distracting leaves and colors. Because if we try to change our entire Life (dealing with the Forest), we will just lose our shit and quit. It's too great, and it's too hard, and well . . .

Take a deep breath—here comes the reason:

We don't see, can't see, or refuse to see. It may or may not be our faults—this blindness—but regardless, we have been lied to and told that we are deserving of Happiness all the time and anything that is hard can't make us that happy. So we quit quit quit and then consider ourselves losers and quitters like the Other People always said we were: *You will never be* _____. Or if they didn't say it, they showed it with their inactions or actions. We fell into the trap of the unconscious parent, the unconscious world—and we became unconscious.

So we agree with that now insidious (spoken or unspoken) Core Belief that we are *less than*, or worthless and quitters, so then we step into that role and live it, buy the story and *read loudly from the Script! Altogether now!* Let's ignore the Forest, look at and fuss with the Trees, repeat it, and never get any Life overhaul at all. No change. No anything. Just Nonsense. Lather. Rinse. Repeat. Life is about balance, right? *Ugh.*

Whew. And also, yeah.

So. We must figure out the biggest obstacle—this One Nonsense Thing—the unique biggest issue standing in our way currently. The One Nonsense Thing is what is causing the vast majority of our own personal suffering, problems, and sticky-stuckness. No matter what brands of Nonsense you have, it is likely that One Nonsense Thing is the pillar of *all* of them, holding the rest of your potential at bay. It is the foundation that the Nonsense house is built upon. It is the framework for failing to reach and achieve our greatest HHS. The One Nonsense Thing is the current, most acute problem, and we must try to overcome it—*forever.*

The One Nonsense Thing is causing suffering. And I know you are suffering. We all are.

This One Nonsense Thing is always the lurker. It will forever be our main issue—if we do not step out, bravely, and decide *No more!* If we do not take a stand and say, *This. Must. Change.*

Then once you identify and deal with the One Nonsense Thing, you might find another.

In his book *The One Thing: The Surprisingly Simple Truth Behind Extraordinary Results*, Gary Keller writes about the importance of focusing on "the one thing" that matters the most to our productivity and accomplishments. Instead of thinking of the One Thing in terms of things we should *do*, like Keller urges, we must look at the One Nonsense Thing differently. This One Nonsense Thing is a poison. It's the crux of your suffering. The One Nonsense Thing is the thing that we must *not* do, we must get rid of, or we must get *out* of our Lives.

I'm not talking about deep childhood stuff here, though that might be where it takes you down the road. (I never said this would be easy. Or did I? I'm sorry). Look, I'm not even talking about effectively blaming. I'm talking about you getting real with your current shit and taking a good hard look at this question:

 What is the biggest Nonsense RIGHT NOW standing in the way of my Health, (pursuit of) Happiness, and Success?

After you answer that question, I want you to think about it. Is the item you just cited the biggest brand of Nonsense in your Life? Or is that a *symptom* of a greater issue? Are you ignoring the Forest? Too many Trees?

Are you overweight because you drink too much and then eat entire pizzas like I did? Do you drink too much because you are exquisitely lonely? Are you lonely because you choose porn over real-Life connections with real people? Do you feel completely unseen in your relationship? Do you get run over, taken for granted, and treated like a mini-butler and short-order cook for your children? Do you hate your job? Do you smoke weed all day long because you don't want to feel a damn thing?

Right now, it doesn't matter if this is your Life story exactly, and no judgments if it is.

But I can assure you that the actual crux of the suffering you are experiencing isn't your bodyweight or your boobs.

Maybe it's your marriage or relationship, or addiction, or relationship to your children. Or the job—the way the job impacts you. Or the deep, dark wound from childhood—that gift that keeps on giving. Which is the number one Nonsense in your Life? The drugs, the relationship, or the job? Or something else? Something deeper?

That is the culling that must happen.

Start with this question:

 What is the biggest Nonsense RIGHT NOW standing in the way of my Health, (pursuit of) Happiness, and Success?

Then ask of your answer, Is it true? Yes or no. Can I peel back more? Is there more Truth? Am I even on the Truth Onion? Peel.

If no, keep asking the question, over and over again:

 What is the biggest Nonsense RIGHT NOW standing in the way of my Health, (pursuit of) Happiness, and Success?

Test your new answer again: Is it true? Yes or no. Peel.

If this is all too hard and you are sitting here with your face in the sand, screaming, "These are all lies" or "I can't freaking do this," then just take a breath.

You can.

You must.

You will.

Peel.

These are not lies. This is the Truth Onion! Like any onion, it stinks and can make you cry. But if it feels hard, remember you are in the putrid, glorious process of changing your Life. Who promised easy or Happy? Not this gal. Also, you can do hard things.

I also did not promise that this would make sense or happen quickly. Like I said, I was sure I had peeled my Truth Onion down to the core—and days before the final draft of this book was due another onion appeared. It's scary. Yes.

But if you are shutting down on me, then let's back up and start with this: Health. What Nonsense is standing in the way of your Health?

Because at the end of the day, our Health is the priority. Without Health, we are suffering—or worse, dead.

Keep going.

Keep peeling until that answer to the second question (Is it true? Yes or no.) is a wholehearted "YES. Yes. This is the One Nonsense Thing. This is in my damn WAY."

Even if that yes feels like a whimper, not an exclamation, even if that whimper feels impossible to tackle, when you know, you know.

The One Nonsense Thing.

And just like that, you have a starting point for the rest of your amazing Life. This is where the Whole Life Overhaul begins. It took me nearly a decade to cull down my Whole Life Overhaul to the simple process of change, to deal with my Nonsense:

Don't drink today. (My One Nonsense Thing.) Fuel your body with food that nourishes it. Get rid of the profession that is crushing your soul. Work on meaningful relationships. Be present for your children. Lift some weights—it makes you feel good and strong. Be a Bear, you badass bitch, and shoot for your biggest Dreams. Go get that book in the library. Be an athlete. Be a best-selling author. But whoops—deal with this new Truth Onion that just sprouted up. Oh well, you've done it before, you can do it again. Peel. You can do that too. Keep going.

This process started with the false belief that the size of my belly was my whole "problem." The difference is that I kept peeling—I wasn't convinced that was really the issue. You may not be convinced either. I didn't quit with my belly. So I didn't keep slamming my head into a brick wall forever. But I did slam my head for years.

Look, you are more than welcome, like me, to take a ten-year, frustrating detour to get to the root of the Nonsense, the core of the Truth Onion(s). You are more than welcome to go through the confusing and delayed process of chipping away at this without rhyme or reason. But I promise—I have done that experiment for you already. That process is dumb and long.

With the Year of No Nonsense process, I am cutting out this whole bullshit line of thinking and hoping to make your Life easier. I have done all the self-bullshitting that should be done for the world—no need to experiment with it; it's a time waster. We are all experts at disguising our Truth, our real problems (the Forest), with all the little issues like "do more yoga" (the Trees). But totally do more yoga, too.

I can tell you that everything happened for me once I identified and took action on my One Nonsense Thing. I can tell you the date and time my Life changed 180-degrees (December 12, 2015, 12:33 a.m.). That one Nonsense item was the key that unlocked many, many doors, emotions, perceptions, and more. You may know what my answer was: *Drinking alcohol is the One Nonsense Thing standing in the way of my greatest Health, (pursuit of) Happiness, and Success. Period. End of story.*

(I know that alcohol is not Nonsense for everyone. But I also know that alcohol is Nonsense for more people than are willing to admit it. So there.)

Truth is an onion. Needing to quit drinking was the core of my onion—my True Truth—at that time. That was my One Nonsense Thing—and I was determined to deal with it.

YOUR ONE NONSENSE THING IS . . .

Great change is often preceded by vicious, searing, soul-level pain. *What is your One Nonsense Thing?*

The kind of pain that burns the eyes. The kind of pain that only a fifth of vodka and a few lines of cocaine might numb. (But perhaps that's what got some of us here in the first place.) *What is your One Nonsense Thing?*

The pain-numb-repeat addiction cycle works—we cease to feel, which is what we are subconsciously after. We don't want pain. And if change is pain—who wants that? We've been trying to avoid suffering, after all! Maybe the cycle is not food or drugs, but we have something going on to numb us. *What is your One Nonsense Thing?*

Because a whole host of us are *Frankenstein's-Monster*-walking our way through Life in this manner. All pieces and parts of us seemingly patched together, leaking pain and grunting, feeling like we are hideous and that no one can possibly understand what we have become or love us. What we have become? Have you felt that—woken up one day and not recognized yourself? *What have I become? Who am I? What happened to me?*

But what "happened" had likely happened long before that moment of the realization. It had been building. For me, I thought my pain started in college with a darkness, Zoloft, booze, and a few days in the looney bin (true). I got better from *that*, but I never fully healed. Why? Because I had been cracked for quite a while—since childhood. Childhood was the great wounding moment for me—and my twenty-year dark booze streak was a way to cope with the twenty years prior to that.

Finding my One Nonsense Thing allowed me to breathe and to see. Because I finally surrendered to just how bad the cracks hurt, and it was okay to not only admit the pain but also heal. I was able to give up the drinking. And move on to the next layer of healing.

We aren't actually *Frankenstein's Monsters*. Check.

And we can't fix and amputate and resuscitate everything at once. If you're a first responder on the scene of a tragic accident, you deal with the shredded femoral artery over the broken toe and busted lip. Stop the bleed. Tend to the One Thing that's going to kill that person.

But anything can kill us!

Yep, that's true.

But what in our lives is damn near certain to kill us—actually or emotionally? That's what we ask. That's the One Nonsense Thing. Once you deal with that, look toward the next thing in line. Over and over again, we bandage, bundle, refresh, reassess, and change the things that are causing the bleed. We are suddenly not so bad.

We start here: we meet ourselves exactly where we are. Head out of sand, the One Nonsense Thing bravely and clearly identified, and we move forward.

My One Nonsense Thing was seriously holding me back—just like yours likely is. My drinking was impeding my Life and clouding my judgment. Once I realized how impactful this One Nonsense Thing was, it changed the entire trajectory of my Life. But again, I drank for a reason. I had to keep peeling. The work does not end there.

Maybe you have identified your One Nonsense Thing, but you don't want to do anything else. You may not be ready to touch what is required to change. Or you may have been living all this time unaware that you could answer this question and start to move toward your Dreams.

What happens if you do all this work, identify that One Nonsense Thing, but then decide No no no no no no.

What if the Fear is too great?

What if you fail?

I mean, what happens if you deal with it?

A bigger question: What happens if you don't?

Give yourself the space to process this, well, process.

· · · · · Checkpoint 9 ·

1. Health:
   > What does Health mean to you?
   > Why are those things important?
   > Now think about why each one of those things *became* important.
   > Finally, is each one truly important? Yes or no.

2. Happiness
   > Think about what things you do, think, act, write, say, and project to move forward in your own (pursuit of) Happiness.
   > What things—big and small—bring contentment?
   > In your pursuit of Happiness, what promises to yourself do you . . .
   >> make?
   >> break?
   >> keep?

3. Success
   > What does Success look like to you?
   > What does Health and (the pursuit of) Happiness mean to you in terms of Success?
   > What is standing in your way?

4. What is your One Nonsense Thing? Did you peel down to the core of the Truth Onion? Where did you start with the process, and what did your process to get to the One Nonsense Thing look like? Diagram it.

5. What other forms of Nonsense did you encounter while peeling the Truth Onion down to your One Nonsense Thing?

#HealthHappinessSuccess #TruthOnion
#OneNonsenseThing #YearOfNoNonsense

10

The Whole Life Overhaul

So, OKAY, MEREDITH, GREAT. I'VE IDENTIFIED MY ONE NONSENSE THING! *Game on! I'm going to change everything!"*

Great! And, well, not so fast. You can't change everything right this second.

You must address your One Nonsense Thing right out of the gate if you want to get the Whole Life Overhaul result. And remember, you have to find your (true) One Nonsense Thing. Are you sure you've got it? Take the time to make sure you have peeled effectively and thoroughly.

If you are cheating on your spouse, you may not need a new job; you must figure out what to do about that cheating thing—and *stat*. *Peel*. If you are a raging drinker, you do not need more green juice to fix the situation—you need to stop drinking. *Peel*. And if your job is slowly killing you, then what are your next options: Going back to school? Looking for a new job? Relocating? Marrying someone filthy rich and devastatingly attractive with a private jet? *Peel*. I jest. Sort of. I mean, marrying someone filthy rich and devastatingly attractive

205

sounds awesome—but that ain't gonna fix your shitty job. You still have to take action on that particular checklist item.

We can read a million things about the benefits of taking small, consistent steps to effectuate major changes. That is all true. But creating a Year of No Nonsense is a complete Life revolution, one Nonsense plucking at a time. And strangely, it doesn't take nearly as much effort as you might think. Because when you are working on the One Nonsense Thing, you are also opening your eyes to all the smaller Nonsense that is also around you. It becomes easy to spot: once you know Nonsense, you know it. The small Nonsense is easy to swipe away. While dealing with the big One.

When we can categorize a behavior or habit, person or place as Nonsense, then we know that we no longer need that drama, lie, or crazy in our lives. We grow stronger and more capable of moving forward, doing what is best for ourselves.

Still, identifying and working to rid yourself of the One Nonsense Thing is the greatest bang for your buck.

Again, you can take the ten-plus-year detour if that's what you want. Not deal with the One Nonsense Thing. But I promise you, removing, changing, or doing whatever is necessary to it will reap huge dividends. Huge. And fast. And once that is out of the way, look at the next One Nonsense Thing—or the next Truth Onion—and attack it the same way.

We want quick results in our culture. We want quick fixes and results—NOW. Here's the great news: identifying and dealing with your One Nonsense Thing is the quickest fix you will *ever* encounter. You will change things *now* if you identify the correct One Nonsense Thing. Read that again. This *is* the quickest Fix.

Oftentimes we try to change a bunch of minutiae and expect these quick, Life-changing results. If we would simply deal with the One Major, Destructive, Soul-Searing, Soul-Sucking, Health-Depleting Nonsense Thing that we have going on right now?

Well, we'd have the Year of No Nonsense snowball effect.

For me, yes, it started with quitting drinking. With quitting drinking, my depression cleared within a few weeks. Truth. I was able to sleep and rest. I cared more about my Health—because I simply felt better. *When you know better, you do better.*

As I felt better, I had the courage to ask for more, to do more, to demand more of myself. To think about a career change. To evaluate my worth and my role in some messes. To consider the relationships that I needed to hang on to and the ones that I needed to let go of. To finally turn the corner to deal with the great wound—the one I uncovered with my new Truth Onion. I am still on this quest—and will likely remain so.

In other words, this is a Lifelong practice.

The Year of No Nonsense becomes a Lifestyle—the Life of No Nonsense.

YOU CAN'T FIX EVERYTHING AT ONCE

Pssssst—you aren't broken.

"Fixing yourself" implies that you are broken. If you are broken, then perhaps you are unable to ever be fixed? You are trash? You are headed straight for the dumpster? (Where you can find the best lasagna!!)

When we feel broken, so many changes are required that it seems like it's better to just chuck ourselves into the landfill than try to fix ourselves. Our "need to fix" list is endless. We then find ourselves in analysis paralysis—and we are stuck. Or even if we think there is Hope, the requirement for change is just too great: *Where do I start? How do I know that's the right place to start? Okay, I did that. Now what?* Finally, this type of "broken" mentality leads to a greater problem: deep despair, depression, and suicidal thinking. *I am broken. I cannot be fixed. Therefore, I cannot go on.*

But the idea of fixing ourselves gives us a sense of satisfaction—until we declare that we aren't fixing well. Then we self-seed ourselves in the "I suck" failure loop.

Repeat after me: I am not broken, and I don't need fixing. (But I got a thing or two that needs some work.)

By choosing to focus on the One Nonsense Thing and continuing to address Nonsense as it evolves, we eliminate the possibility that we are wholly broken. *It's just this One Nonsense Thing, after all.* We zone in, focus on that one thing. We can see the whole picture, because it's this one thing in the way. We can breathe because we aren't paralyzed by all the requirements to change, to try to unbreak, all the Fear inside. We focus on changing that one Nonsense part. Because, well, if it's just this one thing to work on, then we can't be completely broken.

Focusing on what you *can* do—this One Thing right now—is everything. (And you can.)

THE STAGES OF CHANGE: IN A TINY NUTSHELL

When I realized that I truly had a problem with alcohol, I could not "unknow" it. *Awareness* starts change. When you are aware of True Truth—good or bad—it tends to stick with you. But sometimes we also "know" some things are to be avoided; yet we put our hands back into the flames. Because even when something hurts, it might be fulfilling a need in our Life—for excitement, certainty, significance. Awareness is a place that, once reached, cannot be abandoned. Once we are aware, we are awakened about whatever particular issue is before us.

And Awareness, like Truth, is often that *terrible*, stinking, multi-layered Truth Onion.

Most of us, at some point in our lives, have come across the Transtheoretical Model[1] (TTM), also known as the Stages of Change

Model. I find it helpful when I am not only helping *others* but also calling Nonsense on my own stupid or destructive behaviors.*

TTM can be summed up as follows: when we are *ready* to change, we *change*.

A slightly longer summary of the TTM. There are six stages of change. TTM is like a circle—we can return to a prior phase at any time. This is a helpful read to identify where you are, right now, on the One Nonsense Thing.

Precontemplation Stage
(Translation: The Shit-Show Autopilot)

In precontemplation, we are unaware of the troublesome Nonsense or its consequences. Our heads might be in the sand about it, or we truly might be unaware. Key: there is no intention to take action with regard to the troublesome behavior.

Contemplation Stage
(Translation: I Might Be Interested in Changing)

For those of you just coming to the One Nonsense Thing, this is perhaps where we are. Contemplation. Even with this recognition of what needs to change, we may still feel hesitant about correcting the Nonsense behavior(s). We are, in essence, *contemplating* whether we want to change or not. For me (in this stage), I felt the push and pull of drinking to be a completely 50/50. I was equally in need of being a drunk as I was of being sober. *I should quit. I don't want to quit. I should quit. I like to drink. I hate feeling this way. I should quit. I like to drink.*

---

* The criticism of TTM arises mostly in drug addiction, where individuals may truly want to quit, but their drug of choice is so powerful and has caused such destruction with the chemicals in their brains that it feels, becomes, or is potentially dangerous to quit—at least without help. Otherwise, TTM seems to stand the test of time, and I find it helpful for this book.

Preparation Stage
(Translation: I Will Prepare for the Change)

Here, we are prepared to take action toward change. The preparation phase might be the place we park the longest. It's the scariest part. Toes dipped ever so slightly in the water. Testing out if changing feels right.

You can park here for a long, long time—vacillating between preparation and contemplation (I know I did). Remember, the TTM is a circle—we can get on or off at any time, in any phase.

For example, when we are thinking of breaking up with the partner who is hurting us, maybe we vascillate, but we are taking some preparatory steps toward ending the destructive relationship. With binge eating, maybe we go grocery shopping and check out what is around the perimeter—maybe picking up a few healthy foods to try so we don't have crap in the house to trigger binges. Even though maybe we order pizza and drink beer that night. Some steps have been taken toward change.

This phase is where the magic happens.

So many of us are made to believe that we will fail. When we take these small preparatory steps, no matter how tiny, we are saying, "I want more. Even if I fail, I want to try. I will try."

That's it: *I want more. I want less Nonsense. I want more good, less Nonsense.* The belief that something more is available is a huge step. In preparation, the belief that we can have, be, and do better is beginning to take hold.

Action State
(Translation: We are DOING SOMETHING!)

This phase is where you do the things! You take steps to crush the One Nonsense Thing, fully intending to carry through. I am doing things! I am amazing! This is the honeymoon phase. *Can I make it last?* And that is where the struggle lies.

(This is where we often "fail" and end up back on the wheel at contemplation or preparation. Remember, circular trajectory. But I take exception to the term "fail"—more on that later.)

Termination Stage
(Translation: We Have Arrived at Our Destination)

Finally, the termination phase is where we "have no desire to return to [our] unhealthy behaviors and are sure [we] will not relapse."

"Termination" can sound scary. Think of it as, well, a terminal, terminus—a point of departure as well as an ending point. Basically, this is where we want to end up when changing our not-so-great habits or actions. We want to terminate the Nonsense.

Here's What Happened to Me

The infamous get-your-shit-together note on the counter came in 2014.

Fast-forward a year later: I had finished IRONMAN Louisville and was "healthier" in a sense, but I was training a lot, and I had picked up drinking again—and heavily. Over Thanksgiving, I stayed home while the family traveled because I had the flu.

I knew that I was getting older. I knew I was tired. I got darker and darker. I had been here before. This place was familiar. And I got scared. I was back to thinking about driving myself into the tree— often. That scared me even more. (Contemplation.)

I knew that I was not going to make it. I had this foreboding sense that I was going to die within the year. I knew that internal voice was a real threat.

When the family came home after Thanksgiving, I was so very tired. I was tired of feeling the dread of each day, the weight of my own self-inflicted weight, addiction, destruction, and pain.

On December 8, 2015—my husband's birthday—I got extremely drunk. I don't remember what we did or why. Well, that's not true.

There was a striptease involved, and I was apparently the star. I don't dance or strip, for the record. The next morning, his shirt had no buttons, and I hurt in places that indicated that I did—in fact—get super bendy. Sounds like a fun time, right? Sure. I guess it probably was for him.

But I remember none of it and woke up feeling like I was going to lose my mind. *Yo-yo up, yo-yo down.* I couldn't take it anymore. The sheer fact that I had danced was enough to sober me up. I don't dance—not now, not ever. I'm like a newborn giraffe on a dance floor—and I did a *striptease? Was there music?*

I was so embarrassed.

I made the decision that after the holiday party at my husband's job—coming up in four days—I would quit drinking. For good. I knew in my heart that I was quitting—forever. I did not hit rock bottom. I was not hospitalized, arrested, or in an accident. I did not fail to meet a deadline. I did not embarrass myself (that day) at the kids' school or at another event. I only danced—buck-ass naked.

But as Lisa F. Smith, author of *Girl Walks Out of a Bar*, states, "I was circling the drain."

A striptease indicated circling the drain for me. I knew it.[2]

I told my husband, "I am quitting drinking." Even though I know he was somewhat relieved, he said, "Okay. But forever?" (Preparation.)

I said, "Yes. Forever."

He shrugged, "That probably wouldn't be all bad."

Interestingly, the loss that he would experience in losing his drinking buddy was bigger than we both thought. People are impacted by your shitty habits; they're also impacted by the lack of those habits. Lots to adjust to with change. So with my decision to quit, there was no fanfare. No drama. At the party, I figured I would drink a lot—after all, it was my last hurrah.

But I didn't. I was almost cautious. I had already decided to quit. To me, it was done. (Action. Or, Inaction, really.)

Has it been easy to be sober? That is a resounding *hell no*.

That's why the Year of No Nonsense saved me. I came to a place of termination for many things in my Life. I looked at things in *black and white*, Nonsense or not, and I acted on them.

But *Life isn't black-and-white*, you might say—and I did, in fact, say that earlier. We do have room for paradoxes, but not, I would argue, on the damaging things.

The One Nonsense Thing may need to be approached with more of an eye toward black and white. After all, isn't it? Aren't there choices that are yes and no, true or false, good for us or not? Isn't the gray—on certain Life-damaging things—what gets us into trouble with our HHS?

The key component to resolving the One Nonsense Thing—and, as such, the subsequent Whole Life Overhaul and all the onions requiring peeling—is believing that you will not fail. I believed in my heart that I would not fail. I believed that I would quit.

How do you get there? How do you believe? Is belief and certainty all it takes to get to termination? There is no magic pill or bullet to get someone to termination. You have to find the way to terminate Nonsense in the way that works for you.

Termination requires the final Grit and determination that we have inside us. It represents the ultimate want, need, and declaration of our decision to _____ or not to _____. It demands the *passionate persistence* to change this One Nonsense Thing. To get on with our true self—to Live our best Lives.

So even after I quit drinking, I still had Nonsense to uncover. I had a new One Nonsense Thing. It's a lifelong task—this quest.

SELF-LOVE AND SELF-HATE: BOTH ARE A LITTLE BS

When someone is struggling and the advice given by whatever guru of the day is "You should love yourself" or "You should learn to accept yourself as you are," I cringe.

Because that is the single-most useless piece of advice I have ever heard. That's not advice; it's a judgment.

Worse than that, it's harmful and potentially a lie that we begin to tell ourselves. (As discussed in Chapter 4.)

If someone is in pain due to their self-image, body image, or Life in general, then there is a huge chance that they have no earthly idea how to love themselves, how to care for themselves. How the hell does someone wake up one day and say, "I feel pretty. Oh so pretty!?" Or say, "Today I will self-care for this body I hate!"

Not only that, but sometimes you just need to wake up and deal. You don't need to light a candle and take a bath. You need to put on the shitkickers and go to war on your One Nonsense Thing.

What about acceptance, someone asked me recently. "Don't we need to accept ourselves in order to move forward?"

Well it depends on your definition of acceptance.

I mean if you ask Navy SEAL, record holder, and ultra-everything author David Goggins, he would say you don't have to accept shit about yourself or your perceived limitations, but you do have to accept the Truth of who you are, what is real, and what you are doing.[3]

So often it seems that we are forced to "accept" the concept of "acceptance, not Truth. Truth we avoid like the plague."

I just want to be clear that there is a distinction between acceptance and complacency. There is a difference between accepting what is true—at this moment—and accepting it forever. Change what you want—a "little careful kindness goes a long way, and judicious reward is a powerful motivator."[4] Goggins coined the concept of the "accountability mirror"—that we have to look at ourselves for the Truth of what we are, even the ugly. When we are honest with ourselves and how we're actually showing up in the world, we can enable ourselves to do great things. If we're not living a Life that's true to our values— or if we need to restructure our values and beliefs, even—then we have to own up to that. If we show up one way to Other People but another way when we're alone, we have to own up to that as well. We have to align our attitudes and behaviors with our values and who we truly aspire to be.[5]

So sometimes I have a hard time with the "accept and love yourself" mentality, because it seems that we do not leave room for change or growth with that mindset. I like David Goggins—because he does not lean on self-love and self-care as a cure-all. He leans on Truth and work and change—and where applicable, acceptance.

A path to self-love exists—don't get me wrong. But a lack of self-love and self-care is not your One Nonsense Thing! It may be a smaller Nonsense thing, but a million bucks says that's not your One Nonsense Thing right now.

The path to self-love is the *result* of getting rid of Nonsense, particularly the one or two things that are the biggest obstacles to our current Lives. We make a better Life by carving a world and path for ourselves where we *can* love ourselves, where caring for ourselves doesn't feel like a giant leap. Self-love and self-care are a result, a gradual by-product, of a Life with less Nonsense. We clear the Nonsense and thus *make* room for self-love and self-care—*then* it grows.

A Life with less Nonsense turns into a Life capable of more love, acceptance, and care. You make room for the love. You have some shits to give. For some of us, that self-love journey is a long freaking hike for a long freaking time. The self-love and self-care might as well be a spaceship to Planet Ice Cream.

I agree with Jordan B. Peterson's assessment where he writes, "You have some vital role to play in the unfolding destiny of the world. You are, therefore, morally obliged to take care of yourself." So you need to work on clearing the Nonsense, and pronto, so you can get on with this self-care biz.[6] A Nonsense-clearing mission in my Life has led to more self-love, more self-care—and it will do the same for you. I still wake up and hate myself and everyone in the world on some days. But I have tried to ensure that I am not adding Nonsense to my Life. That my Truth is open and available and that I can't pull bullshit on myself, the Other People, or my Life.

As I write this, the time is 4:24 a.m. I am drinking coffee with coconut milk and a side of water with sea salt and lemon. I am wearing socks I love. I practiced a quick moment of gratitude in my journal. For me, this is a major win of a morning.

Why? Because I didn't drink yesterday.

Because I didn't fight with my husband or with anyone on social media.

Because my lunch and dinner yesterday were colorful—green, red, orange—not brown.

Because I slept six hours, not four. (I still need help on the sleep front).

Because I woke up to *write this book*, not sit in traffic with a sugar coffee, a sugar scone, and a sweet-ass case of road rage while dropping off my children, whom I should have been so grateful for—but who annoyed the living hell out of me. Working toward and Living Life.

My Life today is different from before.

But it took time. I didn't wake up and "have this"—I woke up and realized I couldn't have anything I wanted at the clip I was going. And I got to that point by asking myself the Truth. I got to that point by getting rid of Nonsense—by taking the One Nonsense Thing by the horns and saying, "NO!"

Then, and only then, was I able to clear the path to practice all this self-love and self-care in the wee hours of the morning.

STOP THINKING: JUST DO (WELL, SOMETHING)

After you know that you want something (or don't want something anymore), then quit analyzing it. You have decided. Let it stay that way.

We retract our decisions—even ones that are beneficial to us—when we get scared or are feeling large bouts of shame. At some point we want, we decide—and then we slip and slide because of these reasons. We are not weak. Our decision is not necessarily "bad"; rather our resolve is a little rough, unused. We are stretching new muscles. Keep stretching—you have decided.

Keep this promise to yourself. You have found the One Nonsense Thing. Don't talk yourself out of it.

We don't get over a habit or addiction by simply stopping doing or using. We are doing these destructive or self-sabotagy things for a reason, so often the recovery from them is way bigger than just stopping that action. We actually recover by creating a new Life, new desires, and new focus points that make it easier to not fall back into the same patterns. If we don't create a new Life, then all the factors that brought us to addiction in the first place will catch up with us again—and the cycle begins.

In the movie *Beautiful Boy*, there is a scene where the son is speaking about addiction. He is talking with a counselor and (paraphrased) says, "I'm an alcoholic and a drug addict."

Then someone says, "No. That's just how you have been treating your problem."

The One Nonsense Thing might be the way you are treating the real, deep problem. That's why you have to peel to that thing—and then perhaps you solve that but find another Truth Onion. Your One Nonsense Thing might be causing massive destruction, and you do need to stop it—but that doesn't mean you have reached the core.

This is an action-oriented process. Yes, it requires navel-gazing and thought. But it requires true Grit and action as well.

Hillary Biscay (two-time Ultraman champion) once told me during a training session, "Why don't you stop thinking so much about what you need to do—and just do it?" (I think Nike also said something like that.) From training with Hillary, I learned that we are all capable of pushing ourselves beyond where we are. We *all* have more inside us than we believe. David Goggins would say the absolute same. So would any other athlete or entrepreneur or world changer. We simply have more inside us.

But it's not about talking—ever. It's about doing. Action. Not thinking. Action. Action. Do. Do not. Move. Go. Gooooooooooo.

Aha. The script again. *Don't sit there and read it. Tear it up. Change it.*

What *action* can you take? Right now, what can you do, what can you change—what steps will take action on the One Nonsense Thing? Look at the One Nonsense Thing: What steps move you in the direction to "create the Life" that you need or want with regard to ridding yourself of this thing? Envision the power of your Life without it. Envision how you feel without it. Envision the pride you will feel when you have conquered this One Nonsense Thing and moved past it.

About alcohol, I tell people in recovery that my biggest tool for not drinking is to "not make eye contact with a drink." I ignore booze like that one gal at the gym you're always trying to avoid. *Don't look at her, don't look, don't look.* When I am at dinner and someone else is drinking, I don't look at it. I don't smell it or see it.

I know my Life is better without booze, so I focus on that Truth. It's easy to focus on what we don't have (grass is greener mentality), and with the One Nonsense Thing, it becomes easy to fantasize about the good ole days when we did or had xyz. *Oh I wish I could have just one glass of wine (which was ruining my Life)! I wish I could spend one more night with Bob (the man who assaulted me)!*

Stop it. We must remind ourselves how freaking terrible, destructive, and HHS-harming this One Nonsense Thing is. *Wine almost destroyed you! Bob hurt you!*

Do not romanticize the monster. The monster is a monster. Remember that.

Much in the spirit of taking "one day at a time," take one action against your One Nonsense Thing. For me, I took action not to drink each day, each hour, each minute. You may say that not drinking is technically inaction, but anyone who has overcome booze knows that not drinking is an action—it takes deliberate words, power, movement, and strength to *not* drink.

If you want to change your Life, you need to actively seek, find, and accept help. Maybe that help comes not from someone but from something—a book, podcast, journaling. *Resources.*

Don't expect someone to help you if you don't ask.

Stop waiting for the Other People to help you.

You are not their responsibility! You are yours. They have their own Nonsense to deal with. When you sit there thinking they should be taking care of you, you are avoiding your One Nonsense Thing. If we all wait on each other, nothing will ever happen. Because humans are selfish. Deal with it. Stay in your lane. Deal with your own One Nonsense Thing. Worry about your role in relationships—not theirs.

If this describes you—waiting on someone else—then you have to get real. No one knows to come looking for you. No one knows to convince you to change your Life. No one is coming, y'all. They don't know you are missing.

This is your moment—to step forward and begin to walk. The moment you step forward and ask for "proof of Life" from Other People, proof of connection, you will find what you need. You have the Resources. What are they? Who are they? Access them. Ask. We. Don't. Ask.

And no, not everyone will be helpful, kind, or receptive. If the first person you reach out to doesn't respond or text back, then go on to someone else. Just because one person says no, don't stop seeking. Before you start any contact, make a list of five or ten people. Do not stop until you have connected with someone. You will connect with someone—if you keep trying. If you give up? Then you probably won't. Connect. Even if it's a virtual friend—like me. If you don't have five or ten people, then you immediately make a list of five places you can physically go to meet five or ten people. Example: a grocery store, Starbucks, church, AA, triathlon club, online groups, book club. Stop making excuses. I mean every time I'm in a grocery store line, folks are the chattiest on the planet—they will totally talk to you. Spark a convo. "Hey, Fred. I notice you have a cart full of bananas and bubble wrap. What's your weekend looking like?" A guy like Fred probably wants to tell you.

Seems silly, but that is how connection works. You can forge a connection with almost anyone—and if not them, then maybe someone they know. It's really magical, actually.

But I am an introvert. Yes, me too. Sorry. Get out there. Remember, no one is coming for you. But they will recognize you when you show up.

When I decided to take action (instead of thinking so much about things), I was able to dissect what was really happening with my Life, with the One Nonsense Thing. Creating the Life first was not what worked for me. I did not know how or where to begin that huge task.

However, stopping the immediate sledgehammer pain (the One Nonsense Thing) cleared the path for the rest. We must fix the current bleed (the One Nonsense Thing), not the stubbed toe (still Nonsense) or shunned invitation (also Nonsense). Again, the current bleed might not be the major core bleed—but you might not be ready to learn that one yet, and the current one might still be killing you. Go with what you can.

The best fix was doing what I could, immediately. *Action. No more thinking.* The rest will fall into place with consistent work.

TICKING OFF THE NONSENSE

Truth is: Life is a giant series of awful comparisons. Like clockwork, we pass judgment immediately—on ourselves, on others. It's the Blink phenomenon—we have our opinions and biases right out of the gate.

At the end of the day, I Live with my choices. But those choices are mine. I must learn the Truth of what is best for me. I need to be strong in my resolve to change—the One Nonsense Thing and what comes with each new Truth Onion. I need to have the right reasons. So, I reiterated in my mind, *Change takes time. True change will be lasting. Be patient. Take your time. It's a long Life if we are lucky. Breathe. Take in the day. Be grateful for the body you have.*

We are often stuck on a thing or two in our comparison culture. It's not the Other People, but it's some part of our shitty story that we keep replaying. It might be the hang-ups or Names from childhood. If someone called us stupid, then we feel gutted when we see someone else succeeding in "smart" ways. If we always wanted to have children but have been slammed with the inability or the loss of a child, then it's living a Life of daggers at every kid on Instagram. We are stuck—and rightly so. Getting past these losses and Names and roadblocks is not for the faint of heart.

What we are stuck on is likely not the One Nonsense Thing we need to first change. Just know that it may be disguising itself as something else. To make the day-to-day bearable is a challenge when you are working through getting rid of or fixing some Nonsense.

So keeping a record of it all is key.

Having a record of your Nonsense lists and your path to changing the One Nonsense Thing is good. I encourage you to sketch, log, and measure all relevant data points of progress and keep track. Write down everything you see, know, feel, and learn—on paper, on your phone, on your computer. Record it on your voice notes or your camera if you don't write. But get it out of your brain and recorded somewhere. (If you don't like to write, do it anyway.)

Progress is wild.

Remember to use your version of Names and Numbers (Chapter 2) to define the progress.

Here's the key: we must take stock and measure our progress. Every damn morsel of it. Sometimes we need a new yardstick to measure. Here's what I mean. If I am only looking at the Number on the scale as proof of my body's worth or proof of change, then perhaps I can write myself off as a massive failure. All that working out, all those triathlons, all that food weighing and more has amounted to very little movement on the scale. If that were the *only measure* of the Success of the last decade of my Life, then I could say I have failed—and big time. But I measure things based on Health markers, measurements, how I feel in my skin, and more.

I clearly have not failed.

But I must pull my head out of the sand, see, and measure everything that I can to get the right data.

When we look at our big hang-ups and the work we are doing with a wide-angle lens, we should be able to find some positives. If there are no positives at all—and I find that difficult to believe if we are truly putting forth effort—then we must work harder. Period. Hustle and Grit are things; we might need to cultivate them. We may need to reach out, tap into our Resources. Find some answers. Ask some questions. Evaluate.

"Well, what if nothing has changed for years?" you might ask.

Nothing changes when we don't take action. Nothing changes when we are beating our heads against the wrong wall. A lack of action will yield an answer of "nothing has changed."

However, the question is, "Have I really given this quest my *best effort?*"

Or perhaps this question: "Have I tried *at all?*"

Maybe not. But wait!

As we discussed earlier, this might not be your fault. Maybe you didn't know about all this Nonsense, the lies, the Names and Numbers that have caused havoc. Maybe you hadn't identified your One Nonsense Thing until *now.*

So things can and will change starting *right now.* You have new tools, new thoughts, new lists and perspectives now. You have Resources and new ideas.

If you haven't given your best effort until now? Doesn't matter. Not even a little.

As long as you are aware of the Truth and where you want to go, then who cares about the past? Getting crazy about perfection is dangerous. That's why body image is dangerous. That's why you must find these other measurements, talk Truth to yourself about what is actually happening, and then do the best you can—every single day. Starting right now with what you know about the Past, the Present, the Nonsense, and where you want to go.

When you know better, you do better. Everyone is doing the best they can.

· · · · Checkpoint 10 ·

1. You have identified your One Nonsense Thing. Where are you with regard to changing this One Nonsense Thing? Are you just thinking about it? Do you have some plans in place? Are you ready to GO?

2. Regardless of where you *are*, identify the next logical ACTION for you in tackling the One

Nonsense Thing. Make a list of ways you can also approach the One Nonsense Thing if this first action doesn't resonate immediately.

3. Make a list of your Resources—including people, books, and things that can help you on your journey—and who *you* will reach out to if needed.

4. What method will you use to track your data and progress? Set it up now. Make your first entry now. Identify how and when you track your data—keep the promise to yourself and do it.

#OneNonsenseThing #StopRomanticizingTheMonster #BeYourOwnSoulmate #NoOneIsComingForYou #YearOfNoNonsense #TheLifeofNoNonsense

11

Roadblocks and Failures:
The Obstacle *Is* the Way

S O HERE YOU ARE.

You have stepped out into this big, scary, and exhilarating "get rid of Nonsense" wide world. You have shown your hand. You have been vulnerable and honest (or you are trying not to be—in which case, go back and reread the entire book one more time).

You're ready to rid yourself of Nonsense, to step into who you are and go forth. You are brave. You are amazing. You got this! You are awesome!

And—you totally get shat on. By everyone and everything. And then you wonder, "Why do I even bother?"

Well, I've been there. But it's the next part—after the being shat upon—that makes or breaks us, that fosters true change.

The Nonsense-ridding journey isn't a one-and-done. It's a forever mission—one that will be a part of our daily routine—like brushing and flossing. Yes, flossing.

There is no wagon to fall off of. Life is a merry-go-round, and at some point you will leap into a pint of ice cream, be the victim of your own self-sabotage, allow that toxic person to influence you, do something unbelievably stupid on a night when you are drunk. That does not make you weak or prove that wagons exist—it simply means that you are human and subject to human things.

And Nonsense, as clearly established, is a big part of humanity.

Recognizing that Life is not one straight line of perfection, that a deep dive into a deep-dish pizza or the casino is not the end of the world, is a key to getting through relapses in our Nonsense judgment.

When I think about all my regrets or past stupidity, I do one thing: *stop thinking about them.* No matter what has happened in the past—whether long ago or recently—it's still the past. Does our past have repercussions? Of course it does.

But I can't do a thing about all the dumb things I did as a drunk or depressed person. I can't go back. I can't undo the stupid. I can only say, "I am sorry. I was acting like a total idiot. But I am not so much of one now. Or at least I try not to be." The past is the past. And if the Other People want to constantly remind me of my failures and mistakes, then those are people who get cut like the bad wood they are.

Everyone makes mistakes. I can't do a thing about what has transpired prior to me taking my Year of No Nonsense journey. Hell, I can't do a thing about what happened *yesterday.* And neither can you. We can only move forward, deal with the consequences, apologize, or whatever.

Again, that doesn't mean that the past doesn't impact us; it most certainly does. We may need to figure out tools and obtain help to cope with that part of it—therapy or professional help. But even then, you need not reside in the past. You can acknowledge that something happened—and choose to move forward.

Forward is a pace, I constantly remind my athletes.

Failure is also a way of Life.

Relapse and failure are, by their very essence, in the past. Wherever we are—right now—can be different. No matter what just happened (like literally—just happened), we can choose to immediately move forward, forgive ourselves (or others), and continue our Year of No Nonsense.

Learning to recognize the Nonsense behaviors and consciously see them? That is the key to stopping the pattern of unhealthy actions that we need to try to move past. At some point, we simply don't *do* those things anymore. But we may need to do the experiment on ourselves several (dozen or hundred) times to prove that we should get rid of x, y, or z.

One of the greatest freedoms that has come with being a sober person is the gift (or sometimes ungift) of memory. I now remember every damn thing that happened the night before. I know if I mean-tweeted—and if I did, it's because that person had it coming. The cloud of escapism and booze is no longer part of my Life. The Nonsense is gone. On the flip side, I am stuck feeling all the feelings and dealing with the consequences of perhaps my past or the emotional turmoil of regret.

But guess what? That's called Living.

It's how we wake up each day and face that challenge—that's part of our *pursuit of Happiness.*

A Truth: Life is full of disappointments, heartbreak, failures, regrets, and wrongs.

Another truth: We make a Life by persevering through these emotions. We make Success by continuing on, when we are tired, upset, and angry. We secure a future by setting ourselves up for as much Health and pursuit of Happiness as we can along the way.

NONSENSE IS MORE THAN A LITTLE BS.

After discovering the One Nonsense Thing, we have much work to do, yes?

Yes.

And it might take a while to work through this One Nonsense Thing. That's okay. But we still have other Nonsense going on in our lives while we are diligently working on the One Nonsense Thing.

Going forward, we simply must recognize that Nonsense is everywhere. Some big, some small. We know what it is—we know our own; we see others'.

We know our One Nonsense Thing.

But if we recognize all forms of Nonsense for what it is—we have clarity, freedom, Purpose, and, believe it or not, a Map for where we are going.

Nonsense—small, big, and our current One Nonsense Thing—is holding us back from our *greatest* Health, pursuit of Happiness, and Success.

We have One Nonsense Thing that is likely causing the most damage.

We start there.

And we keep identifying and working to rid ourselves of other Nonsense—big and small—each and every single day.

Forward is a pace. Let's just keep moving forward.

FEARLESS

Fear is the thing holding most of us back from stepping into our own greatness, potential, and, yes, those Dreams we talked about. Fear is the thing that halts the good streaks, disguises itself as a lack of motivation, and lights the bitter cyclical flame of self-sabotage. Fear is often the exact thing we must face. "Fear is good. Like self-doubt, fear is an indicator. Fear tells us what we have to do."[1]

Often we Fear situations that are far from Life or death, and therefore we are being held back for no good reason. "Traumas or bad experiences can trigger a fear response within us that is hard to quell.

Yet exposing ourselves to our personal demons is the best way to move past them."[2]

The question, too, is, *What are we so afraid of?*

Marianne Williamson says, in her epic book *A Return to Love,*

> Our deepest fear is not that we are inadequate. Our deepest fear is that we are powerful beyond measure. It is our light, not our darkness that most frightens us. We ask ourselves, Who am I to be brilliant, gorgeous, talented, fabulous? Actually, who are you *not* to be? You are a child of God. Your playing small does not serve the world. . . . We are all meant to shine, as children do. . . . And as we let our own light shine, we unconsciously give other people permission to do the same. As we are liberated from our own fear, our presence automatically liberates others.[3]

We can learn the art of Fearlessness from watching children—at an age before they know Fear. They'll jump off rooftops, leap out of trees, run into traffic. Lord knows, it's terrifying to watch. But they are, essentially, Fearless. Because they have no idea what Fear is. As parents, we can raise our children to be Fearless or terrified—depending on how we respond to their acts of bravery.

Negativity bias is a phenomenon in which we trust negative experiences more than positive experiences or other kinds of information. It has a survival purpose traced back to our paleolithic ancestors over 2.5 million years ago.[4] In other words, if someone saw a saber-toothed tiger, they might say, "Shit. Tiger. Mean. Get club. Run." In other words, being positive in that scenario would have meant certain death: "Aw. Cute. Tiger. Pet! Pet Pet!" *Gone. Dead. Eaten.*

The negativity bias was a Life-saving mechanism back then. But now? Well, it's an instinct that doesn't necessarily serve us as well in the modern world.

We need to fight for our right to change—not against it. We need to fight *ourselves* for the right to change ourselves too. We need to be Fearless—somehow.

A few years ago, eight-year-old James wanted a book titled *How to Survive Anything*. My husband and I thought it was right up his alley, because he loves facts—facts about great white sharks, plants, and cottage cheese. My first clue that this book purchase was a tragic idea should have come from the fact that it was sold at Cabela's—a massive hunting, fishing, and outdoor-sports type of store.

About fifteen minutes down the road, I realized that the Cabela's version may have been a little too much "survival of *anything*."

Bear attacks. Tsunamis. Home invasion. Zombies. Avalanches. (It was actually a survival guide. Translation: it was scary as shit and probably had a disclaimer on it.)

Knowing James, I should have known he would be upset by all these survival facts. And yes, pretty quickly he was visibly upset. The bears and avalanches were all too real, all too close. He was upset to the point where he didn't want the book *in the same room*.

We took the book *out of the house* and put it in the garage. We discussed how James need not worry about bears or tsunamis or avalanches. (I mean, you don't need to worry about them, until you *do* . . . but that was not the point.)

But the next morning, I heard the *pitter-patter, jump-jump* of energetic-little-boy feet come hopping into the room. I was standing by the bed, sorting through my workout clothes, and James said, "Uh, Mom. Where's that book? The survive-anything book."

I looked at him. "Um. Yeah, Dad is taking that book back to the store," I said.

"I need it. I want to learn about how to survive *anything*," and he jumped in place, excitedly.

"But you were scared of the stuff in the book, bud," I said. I paused, in case he forgot. "Remember? Um, like yesterday?"

"Yes, I know!" he said. "But I think it's time that I learn to face my Fears!" He jumped, and off he went, pitter-patter, jump-jump.

So the kid headed to school with his survive-anything guide in hand (and ready to scare the other children at school—whoops). James has been somewhat uncharacteristically Fearless since that book. That's not a dig at him, but he and I are the historically "careful" duo in the family when it comes to certain things.

This new "Fearlessness" was because he was armed with facts, with Truth. Taking it further, when he had Truth on his side, he grew as a kid. He found room to be proud of himself in school, to reject baseball, and to pursue his Dream in art when faced with Truth about all those things.

The same holds true for adults. Truth sets us free. We thrive when we have a clear path and feel safe; when we have the Resources to make ourselves proud, we can Dream and go forth.

Here's the thing about cutting out the Nonsense or pursuing our Dreams or whatever we are "afraid" of: if we are in a place of safety* and acceptance and armed with the Resources, there is nothing to Fear.

And if we are not in a place like this? Well, then we should find one.

Well, great. How do I find that as an adult human?

Answer: by creating and building a Life that is as Nonsense-free as possible.

I believe, too, that the antidote to Fear is tapping into and believing in our Resourcefulness. If we are grabbing our greatest internal resources—creativity, ability to love and learn, Dream chasing, Hope,

---

* Safety is a broad term. For example, we can feel unsafe in our bodies from childhood abuse. We can feel unsafe in our homes or jobs from emotional and past trauma. Something as seemingly small as a fender bender at a young age might make us feel unsafe in a car. Everyone interprets safety differently, and the response is highly individualized. Until we find a safe space for us, we may remain skittish—relying on our One Nonsense Thing for comfort, certainty, and a place of sanity (even if it's insanity).

and strength—then we naturally will Fear *less*. A Life believing we are without Resources is where a deep challenge arises.

It's the Resourcefulness that we have inside ourselves that creates our foundation, our drive, and replaces the Fear constantly driving us.

Think about it this way. If we believe in our hearts that there will always *be* enough, what do we have to Fear? If we believe that we *are* enough, what is there to Fear? With these Core Beliefs, it does not matter if we need to find a new job, place to live, or relationship—because we have the Resourcefulness to not only survive but also thrive. We believe that in our hearts.

Noam Shpancer, PhD, author of the novel *The Good Psychologist*, proposes that our solution to Fear (and its accompanying twin, Anxiety) is twofold. He implores us to "get to know" our Anxiety.

"Stop hating on it. Observe it. Approach it. Befriend it. Fear is like a crying baby, to be pacified it needs to be embraced. . . . Feeling like you're out of control does not mean you're out of control. Our Fear system has evolved to protect us. If you can feel Fear, it means that your systems are working."[5]

Most of our Fear responses are coming from things that we simply haven't found a way to normalize yet. We are not accustomed to putting ourselves on a stage and speaking. Or getting in the open lake to swim. Or looking for a new job, a new relationship.

These things are not zombies or bears—yet they might as well be. They are new and scary. Even the word Fearless scares people. But break it down to the roots—it's simply fearing . . . less. We need not be completely Fearless. We simply need to just Fear *less*. To Fear *less*, we must tap into our Resourcefulness and expose ourselves to exactly that which we "Fear."

When I was broken by a hill called "the Big Sister" on my bike—time and time again—what did I do when I trembled at the base of it?

I went up. I fell down a few times, but I eventually rode it—up and down—twenty times in a row one day. Now, I can climb it effortlessly (okay, maybe with some huffing and puffing) completely and utterly without Fear. I know I will surmount it. I also know that if I don't—the worst that will happen is some cuts, bruises, and busted pride.

If our biggest Fear is failure, this means we simply have not failed enough. We haven't normalized the Fear, given it a small feeling. Or maybe we failed one big time and it hurt mega-bad—but we didn't fail enough times to get that muscle worked. In these circumstances, normalize. It's time to put ourselves out there and fail a little more, even a little bigger.

We got this. Seriously.

KILL THE THINGS YOU CANNOT MODERATE

Many times we set ourselves up for failure by thinking we can handle certain people, places, and things. However, those people, places, and things are actually *Nonsense* (to us), and we need to walk away, like, forever.

If you are friends with or under the watch or care of someone who tells you that you can moderate something, maybe you should run from them. No one should tell you how or what you can moderate, including me. Whoops. But because we all are incapable of moderating things that are dangerous to us, it is clear that desperately trying to moderate certain things becomes part of our personal brand of Nonsense.

Can we moderate things? Sure. We can moderate things that don't mean any harm to us. We can moderate kale and salad, volunteer work and church, textbook reading and puppies. Although some puppies are so cute—moderation feels impossible.

Where we mess ourselves up is trying to moderate things that mess with us. If something is catastrophic to us—emotionally, physically, psychologically, relationally—and we try to have a "little piece of it"?

My made-up definition of addiction is this: *continually attempting to moderate a thing that we cannot moderate, despite all damning evidence proving our complete and utter incapability of moderating said thing.*

Russell Brand, in his book *Recovery*, categorizes addiction as "when natural biological imperatives, like the need for food, sex, relaxation, or status, become prioritized to the point of destructiveness."[6]

Finally, a more expert definition: a substance or behavior "for which the rewarding effects provide a compelling incentive to repeatedly pursue the behavior despite detrimental consequences."[7] If we look at addiction in those terms, why in the world would there be any stigma around it? But this definition makes so much sense.

Below is a list of things that I cannot mess with. And by that, I mean, if I do, then bad things tend to happen or I am certain will happen:

- Alcohol
- Drugs/cigarettes/smoking of any kind
- Looking at the social media of people who make me angry, jealous, bitter, or rage-y
- Reese's peanut butter *anything* (the quickest path to a twenty-pound gain for me)

Making the list of our unmoderatables helps us deal with failure (or perhaps learning to fail) and also working to prevent relapse. The unmoderatables should henceforth go on your list as Nonsense (if they aren't there already). Even if you don't always avoid them, you'll at least know they are on the list of Nonsense.

THE ART OF FAILURE

Relapse, failure, and pain are all part of the process of change and growth. Our desperate quest to avoid pain, coupled with Fear, is yet another thing that holds us back. Most of the time our "failures" *are* stupid or small, but we play them over and over, thinking that the same dumb stuff will just magically happen again. But the Truth is, we might never make the same small, dumb mistake again. It's the big ones that we tend to keep making—because the changes or stakes are also so big.

About a year ago, I had a fall-apart fallout so bad that I couldn't breathe. My eyes were swollen, and I felt as if I hadn't rested in years. I hadn't felt this awful since probably a bad booze binge and shingles in 2014.

My mom texted me, "How are you feeling?"

I wrote her back, "I feel like shit."

With the falling apart, I noted the following themes of language running through my head. The internal dialogue went like this:

1. I am a failure, specifically about x, y, and z.
2. I am a failure in general.
3. Specifically, I am a failure at motherhood, writing, love, money, nutrition, CrossFit, running, swimming, yoga, thinking, reading, existing, Living.

In other words, my falling-aparts center on being a failure. And failing at, like, everything.

No one likes failure. Very few of us take it easily. But here's the thing:

Life is just a Failure Battleground.

Where I am today is at the core of my first Truth Onion and starting on my second one. I have peeled and peeled—it stinks—and here is where I have landed: Failure is awesome. Does it feel that way at the time? No way. But is it, nevertheless, awesome? Yes.

FAILURE TRUTHS:

- Failure is the test of who we are and what we are made of.
- Failure reveals our weaknesses (hard).
- Failure reveals our myriad of strengths (yes!).

- Failure is the opportunity to course-correct.
- Failure shows what we do when we are knocked down. Do we get up? Do we keep going?
- Failure—how we handle it, how we plan our next move— speaks volumes about character. If there is no next move, that speaks as well.
- Failure shakes things up and gives us a new vision.
- Failure forces a new plan.
- Failure is Life's free do-over.
- Failing is the biggest gift of all.

Recently, I spent only about thirty-five hours in my atypical state of falling apart. That might seem long to some of you. But I assure you, this is a record rebound.

Failure, in order to be truly beneficial, does require the *rebound*.

One of my athletes, around the same time, was in the doldrums too. I scrubbed her training plan and inserted two weeks of daily one-mile runs and walks. And that's it. With the description: "If you don't have one mile for yourself, then something needs to change."

She texted me, "I need to make myself a priority and damn right I can find time for one mile and eff—if that wasn't an amazing mile at a record pace." I could help her because I had failed. *Failing is the biggest gift of all.* Because I was right there with her—feeling stuck and sad. Because of that, I knew what I could do to help.

Failure often reveals that I need to let some things go. That perhaps I am "failing" because I am not focusing. I am creating diversions. I am procrastinating.

Or perhaps failure shows me that the things I am letting go of are not "failures" at all—but movements forward, beyond, and through. When I let them go, I am progressing.

Richa Chadha asks, "So what?" when she is struggling with something. "What if I fail? *So what?*" Thinking about the answer as a "So what" or "Who cares" or "Do it anyway" puts some things into a clearer perspective and gives us the courage to look forward.[8]

STOICS LOVE FAILURE

"The impediment to action advances action. What stands in the way becomes the way."

This line, written nearly 2,000 years ago in Marcus Aurelius's private diary, was the inspiration for Ryan Holiday's international bestseller *The Obstacle Is theWay*. Not only has this book pretty much attained "cult" status, but it also should be required reading for humankind.

It totally strips away the notion that we all deserve an easy path. (I tell my children, "The obstacle is the way, kids!" all the time. They stare back, blankly.)

Marcus Aurelius was a "Stoic." Stoics are basically the badasses of overcoming obstacles and working through difficulties—and coming out on the other side not only "okay" but freaking victorious.

The Stoic finds a way to flip a negative into a positive (and not in a fake-feeling-positive way, either), find good in the bad, and reap Success from failure. No matter how terrible or apparently undesirable a situation is or becomes, the thought is that we always have the chance to use the situation as an occasion to be or grow into our best selves.

"We don't control when things get hard, but we always control how we respond. We can show patience, courage, humility, resourcefulness, reason, justice, and creativity. The things that test us make us who we are. The Stoic grows stronger and better with every obstacle they face. They rally to every challenge and thrive as a result. So can you."[9]

The Obstacle Is theWay outlines overcoming obstacles as a discipline with three critical steps: "how we look at our specific problems, our attitude or approach; then the energy and creativity with which we actively break them down and turn them into opportunities; finally, the cultivation and maintenance of an inner will that allows us to handle defeat and difficulty. It's three interdependent, interconnected, and fluidly contingent disciplines: Perception, Action, and the Will."[10]

In short, we can

• see things for what they are (Perception);
• do what we can (Action);
• endure and bear what we must (Will).[11]

We easily get bogged down, stuck in our failures, inadequacies, and roadblocks, and deem these the *reasons* for why we can't change, move forward, or heal. *How can I get past this? What can I possibly do now?*

Cue our Resourcefulness. Cue our Positivity. Cue our recognition and work against the One Nonsense Thing. Cue our list of Nonsense. Narrow the focus on what we can control, what Nonsense we can avoid and eradicate. *Perception (Seeing! Truth!). Action. Will.*

By changing our perception, taking action, and using the strength of our internal power, we create our world. We make a place where our own Nonsense doesn't have power over us. Will we have other Nonsense to contend with? Of course. But we know how to handle that as well—through constantly ridding ourselves of our own Nonsense.

We know how to move forward.

We know.

Sure it's scary.

But we still know how.

And because we know, we must.

· · · · **Checkpoint 11** ·

1. What are you incapable of moderating? What are some steps you can take now to set yourself up for Success in the war against your One Nonsense Thing?

2. "Life is a Failure Battleground." How does this statement make you feel? Do you need to re-frame your Fear of failure? Does it make it easier or harder for you to think that failure is imminent or likely?

3. Think of one Success of yours—what failure or failures precipitated it? (Think hard!)

#ModerationSchmoderation #LifeIsAFailureBattleground #FearLess #YearOfNoNonsense

12

Your Year of No Nonsense

THE MAP

I am hopeful that, after taking the journey through this book and through all the Checkpoints, you arrived at your One Nonsense Thing. You have likely identified more Nonsense, big and small, and you are ready for a Map.

By now, actually, your unique Map for the Year of No Nonsense probably not only feels possible but is an absolute.

Your Map is unique—because it takes into consideration your past, your present, and the future you want. It involves your unique brands of Nonsense and your big One Nonsense Thing. But like most things in Life, it's also up to you to do the work, to take the action, to draw and follow your own Map. The Map for the future is about keeping a promise to yourself: a Year of No Nonsense, which is the unlikely path to a Life of less Nonsense, less BS.

The book is a conglomerate of things to think about—things that will likely spark a clear path for your Map—to guide you to reach your goals by embarking on a Year of No Nonsense. Because Nonsense is subjective and we are unique in every way, it is our decision how to make this happen.

The general steps for the Map are outlined below, based off the Checkpoints you have completed.

Remember that this is your Map, your journey—full of your uniqueness. Make it your own—just make that first step and keep stepping, and you'll be on your way.

FILL IN YOUR MAP

Based on the work you put in to Checkpoints 1 to 11, you have created your Year of No Nonsense Map—without even knowing you have done so.

Hooray for happy serendipities!

Let's go through this (relatively quick and painless) mapmaking process now.

Create Your Backstops

A "backstop" in navigation is a certain point where, if you get to it, you stop and go back—because you are about to be seriously lost.

Before we make the Map, we need to set your backstops—points where you may navigate to and you know that you must turn around, get your bearings, pause—for you are heading down a rabbit hole of Nonsense, no-good things, or sabotage.

If you have been journaling and keeping notes and answering the Checkpoints, now it's time to pull out that information. This will be your guide to your personal Year of No Nonsense.

On a blank, fresh piece of paper in a shiny new notebook, on your phone or computer (or whatever floats your boat), write the following things (listed in bold):

BACKSTOPS:
Two things that are going well are:

(Checkpoint 1, Number 1: These are two nice things happening in your Life right now, no matter how small. A grounding place, to remember there is always something good.)

I am _____.

(Checkpoint 2, Number 3: This is the Name you are choosing to call yourself. Your warrior name. *I am a Bear.*)

Two Lie Rewrites:

(Checkpoint 3, Number 2: These are two lies you have been told, and you have rewritten them. Example: I will never be a runner → *I am a runner.*)

These are your first three Backstops. (Leave some room; we're gonna add a few in a bit.)

When you feel that you have lost your way or you want to quit in the Year of No Nonsense, you go back to these first Backstops, read them, and ground yourself in the Truth.

These are parts of your Truth.

You recall two things that are going well, or come up with two new ones.

You remember your Name.

And you look at two Truths to stand up against the lies that might be told to you or floating around in your head.

Write about the process, stay present. Keep leaning, continue peeling.

Create Your Path

Your One Nonsense Thing has been identified. In identifying this, you have revealed your path—because each day, you are working toward getting rid of this One Nonsense Thing. You now have the Backstops to ground you. Now draw out your map—however you see fit—here we go.

Every day the question is, *Am I taking action? Am I working to get rid of (or change, heal) this One Nonsense Thing?*

Every day? You keep your Dream(s) in the corner of your eye. After all, it's the One Nonsense Thing that is our great hindrance in our Life—to a Life with Health, (pursuit of) Happiness, and Success at the forefront. (Checkpoint 8, Number 1: What is your Dream? Yes, really. What do you want to do with your Life? Are you doing it?)

Put your Dreams in a place where you can see them—on your bathroom mirror, your refrigerator, your screen. When it seems impossible to rid yourself of Nonsense, remember the Dream. You got this.

Your Map: It's Easy

You have Resources (Checkpoint 8, Number 3). Remember to tap into those Resources as you go. The more you access what you *have*, the more Resources you will create, find, and conjure. Your resources open new doors.

Your resources are part of your map. Take lies you discover and remember and turn them into rewritten Truths. Add these new Truths to your Map. Resources, check. Truth, check. Make a diagram of your choosing.

Remember what Health, the pursuit of Happiness, and Success mean to you (Checkpoint 9). Add these to your Map.

When you feel hopeless, go back to your Backstops. Then get back on your map: Resources, Truths, and HHS items. Use the Backstops to continually remind you and ground you in your Year of No Nonsense. Use your Map to guide you; keep drawing, keep writing.

Save Your Map, Change Your Map

Your Map is not permanent. It can adjust and change. You can fix your One Nonsense Thing and then start over with the next One Nonsense Thing. You can add smaller Nonsense things and deal with those.

The Truth though?

You have done major work in simply reading this book. You don't even have to follow any Map—though I do think the Backstops are pretty kickass. You have all the power in you to create your own Map, your own Year of No Nonsense. *When you know, you know. When you know better, you do better. Everyone is doing the best that they can.*

Infinity: Just Keep Moving Forward

My forever theme, my forever mantra: *Just keep moving forward.*

Will your Year of No Nonsense have failure and pain? Yes. Will everything be perfect? Not in a million years. Will you fall? Yes. Will you mess up and hurt the Other People? Yes. Will the Other People continue to hurt and disappoint you? Yes.

What can you do in light of all this perceived bad news?

You can *just keep moving forward.* No matter what happens, always keep moving—keep working, Hustle a little, find your Grit, chase the Dream(s)—and remember, forward is a pace. Just create your Map and go.

IT'S YOUR TIME

When I wrapped up my first official "Year of No Nonsense," was all my Nonsense gone? Nope, and I willingly ate too much pizza last night. (Nonsense!)

But I can report this: the more Nonsense I continue to uncover and work through, the more Health and Success I achieve. The pursuit of Happiness is stepping into my Life—showing up to Live. And that is Success.

Because I can delineate where Nonsense ends and begins, I am more certain about my path. With each day, I get tougher, more sure-footed. My circle of friends gets smaller, but my patience, compassion, and understanding grows bigger for those outside my circle. I am kinder, or I am quieter when I can't be kinder.

My plate is clear(er), and I worry less about things that used to bother me. And yes, perhaps my emotions and anxiety still freak me out—but then quickly settle—because I have learned to lean into the anxiety, to feel it, to sit with it. I may have more breakdowns, but this work on myself, on my Life, is some of the best yet. And I remind myself that when the breakdown happens—it's because I am strong enough now to handle it.

Sometimes we have to fall apart, fail, and relapse to see what the Truth is. Like I have said before, we aren't broken. But sometimes we also can't fill our cracks, and we don't need to. They simply are a part of who we are.

What is hard? Rejection. Fear. Unworthiness.

What hurts? Rejection. Fear. Unworthiness.

What else? The Other People affirming our deepest Fears. All Nonsense things.

With my Year of No Nonsense, I made it my personal mission to persevere and thrive beyond the devastation I have experienced—in recent times, with certain people, in childhood, and all the beautiful, worn cracks in between. The Fear of this Year of No Nonsense was greater than I had known. The obstacles were massive—but likewise, the obstacles were the way.

With no more room for Nonsense, we open up the air for a space of Gratitude, power, peace—and, yes, Vulnerability. Shame and blame cannot grow in the light.[1] With these movements away from Non- sense, we are saying, "I am making room for the light."

And sometimes that is all we need: room for the light. Your bulbs are bright.

GO FORTH

In the Year of No Nonsense, the challenge is not to learn to love yourself. It's not to practice self-care. It's not to step into some form of greatness. It's not to meditate, exercise, or eat kale. It's not to start or end relationships or deconstruct your childhood or failures.

Those all might be things to explore and consider—but that is not the challenge.

The challenge is to Live each day as the best version of yourself. To make room for your own light and Purpose for your Life. To do the best you can and accept that you are doing so; to assume the Other People are doing the best they can, too—if not because it's the right thing to do, then because at least they won't drive you crazy.

You embrace this challenge by identifying the Nonsense in your Life—especially the One Nonsense Thing—and working through and past it. You live your best Life by training yourself to spot Nonsense when it shows up. And then, like a SWAT team, knowing exactly how to respond. You learn to prevent the Nonsense from breeding and taking over. You retreat to your Backstops, look at your Map, and reassess when things get nuts. Is this true? Yes or no. With practice as a Nonsense expert, you grow stronger and stand taller and more powerful in exactly who you are—because you can see exactly what is good, what is bad, and what is the Nonsense in between.

By committing to Live your own Year of No Nonsense (year after year after year), you simply take the pledge to be better, to do better, and to step into your Life.

A few months ago, I walked into my bedroom to see a note on my bedside table.

Oh crap. Not another one.

But it was a note from my daughter. Decorated in pink ink and artfully arranged on the table with stickers, stuffed animals, and, of course, a fashionable string of large plastic pearls.

To: Mom, From: Stella

A leader is not the one who does the greatest things. It's the person who gets others to do the greatest. It's hard to "fale," but it's better to succeed.

I have made a mess of many things, but I am also making things right, day by day. I just keep moving forward—a path of less Nonsense, more Life.

I am worthy of Living.

I am not hard to love.

And neither are you. Truth.

Acknowledgments

JAMES AND STELLA—EVERY DAY YOU MAKE ME STRIVE TO BE BETTER. Without you, I would have never had the courage to chase my Dream, cultivate Grit, and practice the art of Hustle. Remember to simply be who you are—without apologizing to anyone for being you. You are worthy of every space you occupy, every place, and all the things you Dream. You are loved—and not only do I love you, but I *really* like you too.

James Atwood III—without you telling me to "get my shit together," I am not exactly sure when (or if) I would have done so. The Atwood Corporation shall always run well with you on the Board. Growing up together—in more ways than one—has been one of Life's greatest honors. It may never be easy, us forcing our way through Life, but it's always an adventure. I love you. Thank you.

Mom and Dad—a lot of the Year (Life) of No Nonsense finds me still processing so much of my childhood, my mistakes, addictions, and failures, as well as figuring out how to be a conscious parent to my own children. This book is a snapshot of a moment in time. I hope I honored the story of my Life, showed Grace, and can be given

Grace as well. This book was hard, because it was the first time—perhaps in my Life—that I fully tried to make myself proud. In writing, I may have disappointed and hurt you, and I am sorry. But also, in writing my Truth, I am on the path to being free. And I hope that I can free others. Because of you, I have a voice, a Purpose—and of course, a Life. For that, I am grateful. I love you.

Papooh, Linda, and Pete—thank you for being such an important part of my Life. To the rest of my family, near and far, blood and marriage—love to you all. Mombow—you are missed.

Thank you: Ansley Sebring—still my best friend and sistah. William Todd Nixon—for allowing me to scream when no one else could stand to listen—and for all your chips. Susan Wintersteen—for being a monumental touchstone in my Life. Robyn Weller—for always being in my corner and in my inner circle. Gerry Halphen—your initial impact continues to make waves. No bullsh*t there. Roger Smith—for planting my writing roots way back when.

For your friendships and random acts of encouragement when needed most during this book process: Beth Morris, Carrie Hanson, Brett Daniels, Nicole DeBoom, Julia Polloreno, Amy Tillotson, Mike Reilly, Dina Griffin, Jessica Gore, Eden Gordon Hill, Lauren Ollerhead, Brent and Kyle Pease, Katy Borders, Melissa Clarke, Kyrsten Sinema, my friends at Klean Athlete. Ben Rocha for your influence on Stella, being a marble jar friend, and for introducing me to Britt Frank . . . who introduced me to Greg Struve—Britt and Greg, you have no idea how important it was to find you both in the fourteen days before this book was complete. Thank you. For Marissa Connors, Tammy Williams, and Judy Newberry—thank you.

For the many podcast guests who changed my Life and parts of my script in sharing your wisdom with others, thank you: Emily Giffin, Amy Dresner, Tony Hawk, Annie Grace, Sarah Hepola, David Leite, Gary John Bishop, Kate Northrup, Lauren Zander, Emily Fletcher, Dr.

Shefali Tsabary—immense, unshakeable gratitude—and always, Bob Harper.

Bridget Quinn and Danielle Svetcov—for the cosmic connection that led me to the incredible Renee Sedliar. Renee—my BEE—a million No Nonsense thank-yous.

For Georgia and Kansas and Massachusetts. I had no idea the places I lived during writing this book take on personalities. I felt leaving Georgia one way, the power of Kansas in another, and Massachusetts—well, that story has yet to be written, but I like the first draft. Is it weird to thank states? Probably. (I do what I want.)

God. Thank you seems a bit of an understatement. I have peace with these pages, because I said my Truth—as it is right now. It is by Grace . . .

For the haters, the trolls, and those cut out of my Life during my Year of No Nonsense and beyond: each time you tried to bury me, you actually planted me, so I am forever grateful.

Resources:
Keep Empowering Yourself

READ

12 Rules for Life, Jordan B. Peterson

A Girl Walks Out of a Bar, Lisa F. Smith

Adult Children of Emotionally Immature Parents, Lindsay C. Gibson, PsyD

Atomic Habits, James Clear

The Awakened Family, Dr. Shefali Tsabary

Blackout, Sarah Hepola

Blink, Malcolm Gladwell

Brain over Binge, Kathryn Hansen

Can't Hurt Me, David Goggins

The Conscious Parent, Dr. Shefali Tsabary

Daring Greatly, Dr. Brené Brown

Drop the Ball, Tiffany Dufu

Loving What Is, Byron Katie

This Naked Mind, Annie Grace

The Obstacle Is the Way, Ryan Holiday

The One Thing, Gary Keller

Tools of Titans, Tim Ferriss

Tribe of Mentors, Tim Ferriss

Recovery: Freedom from Our Addictions, Russell Brand

The Road Back to You: An Enneagram Journey to Self-discovery, Ian Morgan Cron and Suzanne Stabile

Rising Strong, Dr. Brené Brown

Stop Doing That Sh*t, Gary John Bishop

This Naked Mind, Annie Grace

Triathlon for the Every Woman, Meredith Atwood

Unf*ck Yourself, Gary John Bishop

The Wisdom of the Enneagram: The Complete Guide to Psychological and Spiritual Growth for the Nine Personality Types, Don Richard Riso and Russ Hudson

You Are a Badass, Jen Sincero

LISTEN

Armchair Expert with Dax Shepard (podcast)

Finding Mastery (podcast)

Good Life Project (podcast)

On Purpose with Jay Shetty (podcast)

The Rich Roll Podcast

The Same 24 Hours Podcast

The School of Greatness with Lewis Howes (podcast)

Super Soul Sunday (podcast)

Notes

CHAPTER 1

1. "It's an Avocado!," video posted to YouTube by :D, August 22, 2015, https://www.youtube.com/watch?v=wG2-y5Yf1Oo.

2. "Dr. Maya Angelou: Part I and Part II," *Oprah's SuperSoul Conversations Podcast*, January 22, 2018, and January 24, 2018.

3. "Nonsense," Dictionary.com, http://www.dictionary.com/browse /nonsense?s=t.

4. "Nonsense," Thesaurus.com, http://www.thesaurus.com/browse /nonsense.

5. "How Long to Form a Habit?," PsyBlog, https://www.spring.org .uk/2009/09/how-long-to-form-a-habit.php.

6. Gretchen Rubin, "Stop Expecting to Change Your Habit in 21 Days," *Psychology Today*, October 21, 2009, https://www.psychologytoday.com/us /blog/the-happiness-project/200910/stop-expecting-change-your-habit -in-21-days.

7. "Why Is Pluto No Longer Considered a Planet?," howstuffworks, https://science.howstuffworks.com/pluto-planet.htm.

8. Laurel Kornfeld, "Scientists Debate Planet Definition, Status of Pluto," Spaceflight Insider, May 5, 2019, https://www.spaceflightinsider .com/missions/solar-system/scientists-debate-planet-definition-status -of-pluto.

CHAPTER 2

1. Gary Mack and David Casstevens, *Mind Gym: An Athlete's Guide to Inner Excellence* (New York: Contemporary Books, 2001).

2. Maisha Z. Johnson, "What Privilege Really Means (and Doesn't Mean)—to Clear Up Your Doubts Once and for All," Everyday Feminism, https://everydayfeminism.com/2015/07/what-privilege-really -means.

3. Nadine Burke Harris, "How Childhood Trauma Affects Health Across a Lifetime," TED, https://www.ted.com/talks/nadine_burke _harris_how_childhood_trauma_affects_health_across_a_Lifetime?language =en.

4. Darcia F. Narvaez, PhD, "How to Heal the Primal Wound," PsychologyToday.com, https://www.psychologytoday.com/us/blog/moral -landscapes/201711/how-heal-the-primal-wound.

5. Darcia F. Narvaez, PhD, "The Primal Wound: Do You Have One?," PsychologyToday.com, https://www.psychologytoday.com/us/blog/moral -landscapes/201711/the-primal-wound-do-you-have-one.

6. "Shefali Tsabary: The Awakened Family," *Oprah's SuperSoul Conversations Podcast*, March 18, 2019.

7. *The Same 24 Hours Podcast*, Episode 108, "Britt Frank, LSCSW, LCSW, SEP."

8. *The Same 24 Hours Podcast*, Episode 108.

9. "Shefali Tsabary: The Awakened Family," *Oprah's SuperSoul Conversations Podcast*, March 18, 2019.

10. "Shefali Tsabary."

11. "Shefali Tsabary."

12. "Shefali Tsabary."

13. Amy Morin, "3 Important Ways Childhood Shaped Who You Are," *Psychology Today*, https://www.psychologytoday.com/us/blog/what -mentally-strong-people-dont-do/201709/3-important-ways-your -childhood-shaped-who-you-are.

14. *The Same 24 Hours Podcast*, Episode 108, "Britt Frank, LSCSW, LCSW, SEP."

15. "Somatic Experiencing: How Trauma Can Be Overcome," PsychologyToday.com, https://www.psychologytoday.com/us/blog/the-intelligent-divorce/201503/somatic-experiencing.

16. *The Same 24 Hours Podcast*, Episode 108, "Britt Frank: You Are Not Crazy. You Are Not Broken."

17. "Shame," Dictionary.com, https://www.dictionary.com/browse/shame?s=t.

18. Laurie Mintz, PhD, "Healing Body-Shame and Trauma," *Psychology Today*, https://www.psychologytoday.com/us/blog/stress-and-sex/201510/healing-body-shame-trauma-sharing-my-story-heal-yours.

19. Daniel Goleman, "What Makes a Leader?," in *HBR's 10 Must Reads on Emotional Intelligence* (Cambridge, MA: Harvard Business School Publishing Corporation, 2015), 7.

20. Goleman, "What Makes a Leader?," 8.

21. Goleman, "What Makes a Leader?," 8.

22. Jordan B. Peterson, *12 Rules for Life* (New York: Random House Canada, 2018), 161.

23. Goleman, "What Makes a Leader?," 9.

24. Goleman, "What Makes a Leader?," 8, 10.

25. Michael J. Formica, "Core Truths, Core Beliefs and Obstacles to Progress, Pt. 2," *Psychology Today*, https://www.psychologytoday.com/us/blog/enlightened-living/200808/core-truths-core-beliefs-and-obstacles-progress-pt-2.

26. Katherine King, PsyD, "Core Beliefs Create Our Reality: What Are Yours?" *Psychology Today*, https://www.psychologytoday.com/us/blog/Lifespan-perspectives/201902/core-beliefs-create-our-reality-what-are-yours.

27. Miki Kashtan, PhD, "Intention and Effect," *Psychology Today*, https://www.psychologytoday.com/us/blog/acquired-spontaneity/201308/intention-and-effect.

28. Aletheia Luna, "What Are Toxic Core Beliefs? (+ 9 Ways to Transform Them)," Lonerwolf, https://lonerwolf.com/how-to-change-your-core-beliefs.

29. Peterson, *12 Rules for Life*, 62.

30. Patricia Love, *The Emotional Incest Syndrome: What to Do When a Parent's Love Rules Your Life* (New York: Bantam Books, 1990).

31. Claire Obeid, "Leave It. Change It. Accept It: How Eckhart Tolle Changed My Life," mindbodygreen, https://www.mindbodygreen.com/0 -7538/leave-it-change-it-accept-it-how-eckhart-tolle-changed-my-Life.html.

32. *The Same 24 Hours Podcast*, Episode 109, "Gary John Bishop;" May 6, 2019.

33. M. Scott Peck, *The Road Less Traveled: A New Psychology of Love, Traditional Values and Spiritual Growth* (New York: Touchstone, 2014).

34. Peck, *The Road Less Traveled*.

35. "General Characteristics," Get Bear Smart Society, http://www .bearsmart.com/about-bears/general-characteristics.

36. Rachael Peckham, "Identity Anxiety and the Power and Problem of Naming in African American and Jewish American Literature," *Xavier Review* 29, no. 1 (2009): 30–47, http://mds.marshall.edu/cgi/viewcontent .cgi?article=1035&context=english_faculty.

37. "The Mathematics of Weight Loss | Ruben Meerman | TEDxQUT (edited version)," video posted to YouTube by TEDx Talks, October 10, 2013, https://www.youtube.com/watch?v=vuIlsN32WaE.

38. "Measuring Gravity: Have We Finally Cracked It?," Cosmos, July 14, 2014, https://cosmosmagazine.com/physics/measuring-gravity -have-we-finally-cracked-it.

CHAPTER 3

1. Sara Nash, PhD, "The Problem That Comes After Your Drinking Problem," Medium.com, https://medium.com/s/story/leaving-the-herd-ab 6c02560496.

2. "*The Pursuit of Happyness* (2006)," IMDb, https://www.imdb .com/title/tt0454921.

3. Frank T. McAndrew, "Don't Try to Be Happy: We're Programmed to Be Dissatisfied," *Guardian*, https://www.theguardian.com/commentis free/2016/aug/17/psychology-happiness-contentment-humans-aspire -goals-accomplish-evolution.

4. Phillip Moffitt, "The Tyranny of Expectations," Dharma Wisdom, http://dharmawisdom.org/teachings/articles/tyranny-expectations.

5. Jen Hatmaker, *For the Love: Fighting for Grace in a World of Impossible Standards* (Thomas Nelson, 2015).

6. Christine Hassler and Lissa Rankin, MD, *Expectation Hangover: Overcoming Disappointment in Work, Love, and Life* (Novato, CA: New World Library, 2014).

CHAPTER 4

1. Peterson, *12 Rules for Life*, 63.

2. Dr. Joel Hoomans, "35,000 Decisions: The Great Choices of Strategic Leaders," *Leading Edge Journal*, March 20, 2015, https://go.roberts.edu /leadingedge/the-great-choices-of-strategic-leaders.

3. B. Wansink and J. Sobal, "Mindless Eating: The 200 Daily Food Decisions We Overlook," *Environment and Behavior* 39, no. 1 (2007): 106–123.

4. "The Princess on the Pea," H. C. Andersen Centret, http://www .andersen.sdu.dk/vaerk/hersholt/ThePrincessOnThePea_e.html.

5. Dusty Baxter-Wright, "Tess Holliday's Brilliant Response to Criticism of Our Cosmopolitan Cover," *Cosmopolitan*, September 6, 2018, https://www.cosmopolitan.com/uk/entertainment/a23004671/tess -holliday-response-criticism-cosmopolitan-cover.

CHAPTER 5

1. Brené Brown, "Listening to Shame," Ted2012, https://www.ted .com/talks/brene_brown_listening_to_shame.

2. The Work of Byron Katie (http://thework.com).

3. Brené Brown, "'Shame Is Lethal' | SuperSoul Sunday | Oprah Winfrey Network," video posted to YouTube by OWN, https://www.youtube .com/watch?v=GEBjNv5M784.

4. Phillip Moffitt, "How Suffering Got a Bad Name," Life Balance Institute, April 11, 2013, http://www.lifebalanceinstitute.com/blog /how-suffering-got-bad-name.

5. Byron Katie, "*Loving What Is: Four Questions That Can Change Your Life*," The Work, http://thework.com/en/tools-do-work.

CHAPTER 6

1. Brené Brown, *Dare to Lead: Brave Work, Tough Conversations, Whole Hearts* (New York: Random House, 2018).

2. Esther Perel, "Rethinking Infidelity . . . a Talk for Anyone Who Has Ever Loved," TED2015, https://www.ted.com/talks/esther_perel _rethinking_infidelity_a_talk_for_anyone_who_has_ever_loved/transcript ?language=en.

3. Malcolm Gladwell, *Blink* (New York: Back Bay Books, 2014).

CHAPTER 7

1. Sherry Pagoto, "Are You a People Pleaser?," *Psychology Today*, October 26, 2012, https://www.psychologytoday.com/us/blog/shrink/201210 /are-you-people-pleaser.

2. Pagoto, "Are You a People Pleaser?"

3. Pagoto, "Are You a People Pleaser?"

4. Patricia Love, *The Emotional Incest Syndrome: What to Do When a Parent's Love Rules Your Life* (New York: Bantam Books, 1990).

5. Judith Orloff, "The Differences Between Highly Sensitive People and Empaths," *Psychology Today*, June 3, 2017, https://www.psychology today.com/us/blog/the-empaths-survival-guide/201706/the -differences-between-highly-sensitive-people-and-empaths.

6. Linda Babcock and Sara Laschever, *Women Don't Ask: Negotiation and the Gender Divide* (Princeton, NJ: Princeton University Press, 2003).

7. *The Same 24 Hours Podcast*, Episode 57: "James Lawrence: The Iron Cowboy."

8. "*Justin Bieber's Believe* (2013)," IMDB, https://www.imdb.com /title/tt3165608.

9. Scott Wilhite, "Roosevelt Was Wrong, Comparison Is Not the Thief of Joy," *Medium*, March 4, 2017, https://medium.com/thrive -global/roosevelt-was-wrong-comparison-is-not-the-thief-of-joy -9e490cd6225.

CHAPTER 8

1. "List of Problems Solved by MacGyver," MacGyver Wiki, http://macgyver.wikia.com/wiki/List_of_problems_solved_by_MacGyver.

2. *The Same 24 Hours Podcast*, Episode 108: "Gary John Bishop."

3. Peterson, *12 Rules for Life*, 63.

4. "Earl Nightengale," Goodreads, https://www.goodreads.com/quotes/32384-never-give-up-on-a-dream-just-because-of-the.

5. Paul Peace, "A Heart-Warming Story of Resourcefulness," LinkedIn, January 15, 2016, https://www.linkedin.com/ulse/heart-warming-story-resourcefulness-paul-peace.

6. "Resourcefulness," Dictionary.com, http://www.dictionary.com/browse/resourcefulness.

7. Google definition of "Resourcefulness," https://www.google.com/search?q=definition+of+resourcefulness&rlz=1C1CHBF_enUS725US726&oq=definition+of+resourcefulness&aqs=chrome..69i57j0l5.4914j1j4&sourceid=chrome&ie=UTF-8.

8. Angela Duckworth, Grit (New York: Penguin, 2016).

9. "The Ride Home," Changing the Game Project, https://changingthegameproject.com/the-ride-home-after-the-game.

CHAPTER 9

1. Peterson, *12 Rules for Life*, 170.

CHAPTER 10

1. "The Transtheoretical Model (Stages of Change)," Boston University School of Public Health, http://sphweb.bumc.bu.edu/otlt/MPH-Modules/SB/BehavioralChangeTheories/BehavioralChangeTheories6.html.

2. *The Same 24 Hours Podcast*.

3. Rob Hill, "Inspiring Lessons from an Interview with David Goggins," *Medium*, February 10, 2017, https://medium.com/thrive-global/inspiring-lessons-from-an-interview-with-david-goggins-3b774ec90e83.

4. Peterson, *12 Rules for Life*, 95.

5. Hill, "Inspiring Lessons from an Interview with David Goggins."

6. Peterson, *12 Rules for Life*, 62.

CHAPTER 11

1. Steven Pressfield, *The War of Art: Winning the Creative Battle* (New York: Ruggedland, 2002), 40.

2. "Fear," *Psychology Today*, https://www.psychologytoday.com/us/basics/fear.

3. Marianne Williamson, *A Return to Love: Reflections on the Principles of A Course in Miracles* (New York: Harper Collins, 1992), ch. 7, sect. 3 (190–191).

4. "Know Your Brain, Accelerate Leadership Performance!," *Leadership Tangles*, August 17, 2015, http://www.leadershiptangles.com/leadership-tangles-blog/know-your-brain-accelerate-leadership-performance.

5. Noam Shpancer, "Fear Is Nothing to Be Feared," *Psychology Today*, December 26, 2017, https://www.psychologytoday.com/us/blog/insight-therapy/201712/fear-is-nothing-be-feared.

6. Russell Brand, Recovery: Freedom from Our Addictions (New York: Henry Holt and Company, 2017).

7. "Addiction," *Psychology Today*, https://www.psychologytoday.com/us/basics/addiction.

8. The "So What" exercise cited by Richa Chadha in Tim Ferriss, *Tribe of Mentors* (New York: Houghton Mifflin Harcourt, 2016), 90.

9. "*The Obstacle Is the Way* by Ryan Holiday: Book Summary, Key Lessons and Best Quotes," Daily Stoic, https://dailystoic.com/obstacle-is-the-way-summary.

10. "*The Obstacle Is the Way* by Ryan Holiday."

11. "*The Obstacle Is the Way* by Ryan Holiday."

CHAPTER 12

1. Brené Brown, "Shame Is Lethal."

Index